MAIN    RD COSMETOLOGY

# Exam Review

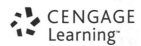

CENGAGE
Learning™

Australia • Brazil • Japan • Korea • Mexico • Singapore • Spain • United Kingdom • United States

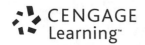

**Milady Standard Cosmetology Exam Review**

Milady

President, Milady: Dawn Gerrain

Associate Acquisitions Editor: Philip Mandl

Editorial Assistant: Maria K. Hebert

Director of Beauty Industry Relations: Sandra Bruce

Executive Marketing Manager: Gerard McAvey

Production Director: Wendy Troeger

Senior Content Project Manager: Angela Sheehan

Art Director: Benj Gleeksman

For product information and technology assistance, contact us at **Professional & Career Group Customer Support, 1-800-648-7450**

For permission to use material from this text or product, submit all requests online at **cengage.com/permissions**. Further permissions questions can be e-mailed to **permissionrequest@cengage.com**.

Library of Congress Control Number: 2010903896

ISBN-13: 978-1-4390-5921-0
ISBN-10: 1-4390-5921-7

**Milady**
5 Maxwell Drive
Clifton Park, NY 12065-2919
USA

Cengage Learning products are represented in Canada by Nelson Education, Ltd.

For your lifelong learning solutions, visit **milady.cengage.com**
Visit our corporate website at **cengage.com**.

**Notice to the Reader**

Publisher does not warrant or guarantee any of the products described herein or perform any independent analysis in connection with any of the product information contained herein. Publisher does not assume, and expressly disclaims, any obligation to obtain and include information other than that provided to it by the manufacturer. The reader is expressly warned to consider and adopt all safety precautions that might be indicated by the activities described herein and to avoid all potential hazards. By following the instructions contained herein, the reader willingly assumes all risks in connection with such instructions. The publisher makes no representations or warranties of any kind, including but not limited to, the warranties of fitness for particular purpose or merchantability, nor are any such representations implied with respect to the material set forth herein, and the publisher takes no responsibility with respect to such material. The publisher shall not be liable for any special, consequential, or exemplary damages resulting, in whole or part, from the readers' use of, or reliance upon, this material.

Printed in the United States of America
1 2 3 4 5 15 14 13 12 11

# Contents

# Foreword

This book of exam reviews contains questions similar to those that may be found on state licensing exams for cosmetology. It employs the multiple-choice type question, which has been widely adopted and approved by the majority of state licensing boards.

Groups of questions have been arranged under major subject areas. To get the maximum advantage when using this book, it is advisable that the review of subject matter take place shortly after its classroom presentation.

This review book reflects advances in cosmetology. It attempts to keep pace with, and insure a basic understanding of, infection control, anatomy, physiology, and salon business applicable to the professional cosmetologist, client consultation guidelines, chemical safety in the salon, and basic procedures as well as some of the more advanced and creative aspects of the profession.

The book serves as an excellent guide for the student as well as for the experienced cosmetologist. It provides a reliable standard against which professionals can measure their knowledge, understanding, and abilities.

Furthermore, these reviews will help students and professionals alike to gain a more thorough understanding of the full scope of their work as they review practical performance skills and related theory. They will increase their ability to evaluate new products and procedures and to be better qualified professionals for dealing with the needs of their clients.

CHAPTER

# 1 History and Career Opportunities

## MULTIPLE CHOICE

1. Which of the following civilizations was the first to infuse essential oils from the leaves, bark, and blossoms of plants for use as perfumes and for purification purposes?
   a. Chinese                    c. Romans
   b. Egyptians                  d. Greeks          ____

2. The ancient _____ were the first to cultivate beauty in an extravagant fashion.
   a. Egyptians                  c. Greeks
   b. Romans                     d. Chinese         ____

3. To achieve a look of greater intelligence during the Renaissance, women:
   a. wore highly colored lip preparations
   b. dyed their hair black or dark brown
   c. wore elaborate, elegant clothing
   d. shaved their eyebrows and hairline           ____

4. During the Middle Ages, women wore colored makeup on their:
   a. ears                       c. lips
   b. hands                      d. eyes            ____

5. In ancient Rome, haircolor was used by women to indicate:
   a. personal wealth            c. marital status
   b. class in society           d. education level ____

6. Archaeologists believe that the practices of haircutting and hairstyling began sometime during the:
   a. Middle Ages                c. Victorian Age
   b. Renaissance                d. Ice Age         ____

7. During the _____, women commonly used henna to add color to their lips and cheeks.
   a. Egyptian era               c. Renaissance
   b. Victorian Age              d. Middle Ages     ____

8. A _____ provides a connection between salons and their staff and the rest of the beauty industry by providing information about new products, new trends, and new techniques.
   a. salon trainer
   b. manufacturer educator
   c. haircolor specialist
   d. distributor sales consultant

   ____

9. In order to get experience providing hairstyling services on film and TV sets, you should be prepared to _____ for a period of time.
   a. work only a few hours a day
   b. volunteer
   c. work without implements
   d. immediately join a union

   ____

10. To be a successful salon manager, you must have an aptitude for math and accounting and understand:
    a. anatomy
    b. marketing
    c. chemistry
    d. physiology

    ____

11. The curling iron was invented by:
    a. Vidal Sassoon
    b. Max Factor
    c. Marcel Grateau
    d. Sarah Breedlove

    ____

12. The innovator who produced and sold makeup to movie stars that would not cake or crack under hot movie lights was:
    a. Noel DeCaprio
    b. Max Factor
    c. Charles Nessler
    d. Arnold F. Willatt

    ____

13. In 2003, _____ introduced the first consumer-oriented DVD to the professional salon industry in order to speak directly to the consumer.
    a. Sebastian International
    b. Max Factor
    c. Vidal Sassoon
    d. Vance Research Services

    ____

14. The individual credited with coining the term *day spa* is:
    a. Sarah Breedlove
    b. Marcel Grateau
    c. Noel DeCaprio
    d. Madam C.J. Walker

    ____

15. The beauty icon who turned the hairstyling world on its ear with revolutionary geometric cuts was:
    a. Max Factor
    b. Vidal Sassoon
    c. Charles Nessler
    d. Queen Nefertiti

    ____

# 2 Life Skills

## MULTIPLE CHOICE

1. Short-term goals are those goals that can generally be completed within one _____ or less.
   - a. day
   - b. year
   - c. month
   - d. week ____

2. Which of these terms refers to the moral principles by which we live and work?
   - a. equality
   - b. emotions
   - c. ethics
   - d. justice ____

3. All of the following are reasons why cosmetologists should study and have a thorough understanding of life skills *except*:
   - a. Having good life skills eliminates the need for self-esteem.
   - b. Well-developed life skills help you deal with difficult clients and coworkers.
   - c. Practicing life skills leads to a more satisfying and productive career.
   - d. Life skills help you keep interactions with clients positive. ____

4. Which of the following is one of the guidelines for success?
   - a. Always strive to meet your salon manager's definition of success.
   - b. Show respect only for those people who can help you in your career.
   - c. Never practice new behaviors.
   - d. Keep your personal life separate from your work. ____

5. Which of the following is one of the recommended strategies for effectively managing your time?
   - a. Make time management a habit.
   - b. Do not schedule free time into your day because free time is a waste of time.
   - c. Always work as hard as possible, even if it means neglecting physical activity.
   - d. Plan your commitments around your leisure time. ____

6. Effective communicators usually have _____, caring personalities.
   - a. clinical
   - b. warm
   - c. chilly
   - d. calculating ____

7. In order to be diplomatic, you should be assertive rather than:
   a. aggressive
   b. intelligent
   c. sensitive
   d. considerate
   ____

8. It is recommended that you study during blocks of time that would otherwise be wasted, such as while:
   a. getting sufficient rest
   b. practicing new skills
   c. listening to your instructor
   d. waiting in a doctor's office
   ____

9. When we pay attention to our natural _____, we can learn how to manage our time efficiently.
   a. insecurities
   b. cravings
   c. rhythms
   d. feelings of guilt
   ____

10. Unfortunately, even if you are creative enough, talented enough, and motivated enough, you will still run into _____ as a cosmetologist.
    a. difficulties
    b. opportunities
    c. friendly people
    d. feelings of guilt
    ____

11. An unhealthy compulsion to do things perfectly is called:
    a. punctuality
    b. procrastination
    c. professionalism
    d. perfectionism
    ____

12. The conscious act of planning your life instead of just letting things happen is described as having:
    a. ambition
    b. a game plan
    c. goals
    d. dreams
    ____

13. The thing that propels you to do something is:
    a. ambition
    b. self-esteem
    c. motivation
    d. professionalism
    ____

14. Putting off until tomorrow what you can do today is called:
    a. time management
    b. procrastination
    c. goal setting
    d. scheduling
    ____

15. Self-_____ involves knowing what you want to achieve and keeping yourself on track so that you do eventually achieve your goal.
    a. esteem
    b. centeredness
    c. involvement
    d. management
    ____

# CHAPTER 3 Your Professional Image

## MULTIPLE CHOICE

1. Your clothing should always be stylish and:
   - **a.** highly accessorized
   - **b.** formal
   - **c.** functional
   - **d.** colorful
   _____

2. An important aspect of professional image is:
   - **a.** physical attractiveness
   - **b.** physical presentation
   - **c.** physical problems
   - **d.** physical activity
   _____

3. The key to prevent repetitive motion injury is to be aware of:
   - **a.** body posture and movements
   - **b.** ill-fitting shoes and fatigue
   - **c.** body manipulation and stress
   - **d.** body vascular system
   _____

4. Behaving _____ includes having a genuine interest in your own day-to-day activities, as well as being concerned about and for others.
   - **a.** personally
   - **b.** politically
   - **c.** politely
   - **d.** professionally
   _____

5. Your back and shoulders should be relaxed and _____ when you are providing client services.
   - **a.** slightly curved
   - **b.** level
   - **c.** slightly arched
   - **d.** extended
   _____

6. Open-toed sandals are _____ footwear when working in a salon.
   - **a.** appropriate
   - **b.** inappropriate
   - **c.** recommended
   - **d.** comfortable
   _____

7. The science of how a workplace can best be designed for comfort, safety, efficiency, and productivity is:
   - **a.** economics
   - **b.** ergonology
   - **c.** ergonomics
   - **d.** ecology
   _____

8. The daily maintenance of cleanliness is:
   - **a.** personal hygiene
   - **b.** physical presentation
   - **c.** professional image
   - **d.** professional hygiene
   _____

9. The impression you project through your outward appearance and conduct in the workplace is your:
   a. personal hygiene
   b. physical presentation
   c. professional image
   d. professional hygiene ____

10. Your posture and the way you walk and move are part of your:
    a. personal hygiene
    b. physical presentation
    c. professional presentation
    d. personal image ____

# CHAPTER 4 Communicating for Success

## MULTIPLE CHOICE

1. People who create conflict wherever they go typically do so because they are feeling:
   - **a.** fatigued
   - **b.** restless
   - **c.** insecure
   - **d.** trustful
   ____

2. In handling a client who is dissatisfied with a service, the ultimate goal is to:
   - **a.** convince the client that you are right and she is wrong
   - **b.** make the client happy enough to pay for the service and return in the future
   - **c.** get the client out of the salon as quickly as possible
   - **d.** fully satisfy the client, regardless of the cost
   ____

3. All of the following are golden rules of human relations *except*:
   - **a.** Being right is the same as acting righteous.
   - **b.** A smile is worth a million times more than a sneer.
   - **c.** Always remember that listening is the best relationship builder.
   - **d.** Laugh often.
   ____

4. Step 6 of the 10-step consultation method is:
   - **a.** Review the intake form.
   - **b.** Determine the client's preferences.
   - **c.** Show and tell.
   - **d.** Discuss upkeep and maintenance.
   ____

5. All of the following are primary criteria to consider when suggesting hairstyle options to a client *except*:
   - **a.** lifestyle
   - **b.** face shape
   - **c.** hair type
   - **d.** hair color
   ____

6. The ability to understand people is _____ to the success of a cosmetologist.
   - **a.** key
   - **b.** irrelevant
   - **c.** incidental
   - **d.** unimportant
   ____

7. To earn clients' _____ and loyalty, you should set aside a few minutes to take new clients on a quick tour of the salon, smile, and be yourself.
   a. money
   b. affection
   c. trust
   d. respect
   _____

8. If a client requests a specific cut or color that she has seen on a celebrity, you should _____ explain whether the look is right for the client.
   a. democratically
   b. diplomatically
   c. directly
   d. distinctly
   _____

9. If you have clients who are habitually_____, it is recommended that you ask them to arrive earlier than their actual appointment time.
   a. late
   b. loud
   c. punctual
   d. unfriendly
   _____

10. When you meet an older client for the first time, it is recommended that you address her with a(n) _____, such as "Mrs. Smith."
    a. honorable mention
    b. honor
    c. honorarium
    d. honorific
    _____

11. It is best to avoid using _____ terms when conversing with clients.
    a. casual
    b. respectful
    c. slang
    d. professional
    _____

12. As a cosmetologist, do not attempt to fulfill the role of_____, career guide, parental sounding board, and motivational coach for your clients.
    a. haircolor expert
    b. counselor
    c. professional acquaintance
    d. polite listener
    _____

13. If, during a discussion, a client is revealing increasingly personal details, it is recommended that you change the subject or _____ to help take her mind off of her troubles.
    a. suggest a mini relaxation service
    b. reveal a personal detail of your own
    c. walk away from the client
    d. turn on a loud machine
    _____

14. You should be open and honest in all of your communications with coworkers, but you must also be _____ to circumstances in which being direct would be hurtful.
    a. oblivious
    b. sensitive
    c. frightened
    d. averse

    ____

15. When you need to speak with your manager about an issue or problem, it is recommended that you _____ beforehand.
    a. cover up your mistakes
    b. think of possible excuses
    c. think of possible solutions
    d. think of who you can blame

    ____

16. The act of successfully sharing information between two people so that the information is understood is called:
    a. direct communication
    b. effective communication
    c. strong communication
    d. overt communication

    ____

17. The document also known as a client questionnaire or consultation card is the:
    a. intake form
    b. welcome form
    c. greeting form
    d. entrance form

    ____

18. The verbal communication also known as the needs assessment is the:
    a. client conversation
    b. client communion
    c. client consultation
    d. client conference

    ____

19. Instead of the term *client*, patrons of day spas are commonly called:
    a. guests
    b. tenants
    c. visitors
    d. day trippers

    ____

20. The term commonly used for patrons of medical spas is:
    a. guests
    b. tenants
    c. visitors
    d. clients

    ____

## CHAPTER 5

# Infection Control: Principles and Practices

## MULTIPLE CHOICE

1. Cocci are bacteria that are:
   a. round-shaped
   b. rod-shaped
   c. flat-shaped
   d. spore-shaped ____

2. Which type of bacteria can cause strep throat or blood poisoning?
   a. fungi
   b. spirilla
   c. bacilli
   d. streptococci ____

3. Bacteria that grow in pairs and can cause pneumonia are:
   a. diplococci
   b. diphtheria
   c. discarded
   d. toxins ____

4. Lyme disease and syphilis are caused by spiral or corkscrew-shaped bacteria called:
   a. flagella
   b. strep
   c. spirilla
   d. cocci ____

5. In 2000, a bacteria called *Mycobacterium fortuitum* caused a client outbreak due to the failure of the practitioner to follow proper disinfection guidelines for:
   a. sharp implements
   b. whirlpool foot spas
   c. shampoo stations
   d. styling chairs ____

6. Bacteria generally consist of an outer cell wall containing a liquid called:
   a. nucleic acid
   b. cytoplasm
   c. protoplasm
   d. protons ____

7. The process whereby bacteria grow, reproduce, and divide into two new cells is:
   a. binary fission
   b. meiosis
   c. photosynthesis
   d. metamorphosis ____

8. The presence of pus is a sign of:
   a. immunity
   b. congestion
   c. bacterial infection
   d. sunburn ____

9. A _____ infection appears as a lesion containing pus and is confined to a particular part of the body.
   a. contagious
   c. primary
   b. local
   d. secondary
   ____

10. Which of the following is a condition caused by an infestation of head lice?
    a. hepatitis
    c. pediculosis capitis
    b. scabies
    d. tinea pedis
    ____

11. The ability of the body to destroy and resist infection is called:
    a. immunity
    c. stasis
    b. decontamination
    d. regulation
    ____

12. Disinfectants used in salons must carry a(n) _____ registration number.
    a. Food and Drug Administration (FDA)
    b. Occupation Protection Agency (OPA)
    c. U.S. Department of Labor (DOL)
    d. Environmental Protection Agency (EPA)
    ____

13. Which agency publishes the guidelines known as Universal Precautions?
    a. FDA
    c. CDC
    b. OSHA
    d. EPA
    ____

14. A salon implement that accidentally comes in contact with blood or body fluids must be thoroughly cleaned and:
    a. completely immersed in an EPA-registered disinfectant
    b. rinsed in an EPA-registered tuberculocidal antiseptic that kills HIV and HBV
    c. placed in an EPA-registered antiseptic that kills HIV and hepatitis
    d. briefly dipped in an EPA-registered solution that kills HIV and AIDS
    ____

15. Disinfectants with a high pH that can cause skin irritation or burn the skin or eyes are:
    a. alcohol and bleach
    c. alcohol and quats
    b. EPA-registered disinfectants
    d. phenolic disinfectants
    ____

16. When washing your hands, you apply soap, lather and scrub your hands and under the free edges of nails with a nail brush for at least:
    a. 5 minutes
    c. 45 seconds
    b. 1 minute
    d. 10 seconds
    ____

17. Antiseptics are effective for:
    a. disinfecting instruments
    b. killing germs on the hands
    c. disinfecting equipment
    d. sterilizing equipment ____

18. Universal Precautions require employees to assume that human blood and body fluids are infectious for:
    a. bloodborne pathogens
    b. nonpathogenic pathogens
    c. influenza
    d. fungi ____

19. Which of the following is *not* part of your professional responsibilities?
    a. follow state and federal laws
    b. keep your license current
    c. check for changes to rules
    d. take shortcuts for cleaning ____

20. When disinfecting a whirlpool foot spa after use by a client, you must circulate the disinfectant for _____ or for the time recommended by the manufacturer.
    a. 5 minutes
    b. 10 minutes
    c. 60 seconds
    d. 20 minutes ____

21. You should clean a whirlpool foot spa and leave disinfectant solution in it overnight:
    a. every day
    b. at least once a month
    c. at least once a week
    d. never ____

22. After cleaning and disinfecting a pipe-less foot spa at the end of the day, how should you dry it?
    a. with a clean paper towel
    b. with a clean linen towel
    c. with a blowdryer
    d. let it air dry ____

23. Which form of hepatitis is the most difficult to kill on a surface?
    a. hepatitis A
    b. hepatitis B
    c. hepatitis C
    d. hepatitis D ____

24. Accelerated hydrogen peroxide, or AHP, is a recently approved form of disinfectant that only needs to be changed every:
    a. 5 days
    b. 30 days
    c. 7 days
    d. 14 days ____

25. It is important to wear _____ while disinfecting nonelectrical tools and implements.
    a. gloves
    b. goggles
    c. an apron
    d. a facemask ____

26. Licensing, enforcement, and your conduct when you are working in the salon are regulated by _____ agencies.
   a. federal
   b. state
   c. city
   d. international ____

27. Some _____ disinfectants are harmful to salon tools and equipment.
   a. antifungal
   b. nonporous
   c. hospital
   d. tuberculocidal ____

28. As a cosmetologist, you are _____ to recommend treatments for diseases.
   a. required
   b. not allowed
   c. encouraged
   d. allowed ____

29. Cosmetologists are not allowed to trim or cut living skin around:
   a. the lunula
   b. the nail tip
   c. any part of the nail
   d. the nail bed ____

30. Fungal infections are much more common on the _____ than on the hands.
   a. ears
   b. feet
   c. cheeks
   d. knees ____

31. A surface must be properly cleaned before it can be:
   a. disinfected
   b. painted
   c. redecorated
   d. resurfaced ____

32. Sterilization is the most reliable means of:
   a. infection control
   b. cleaning
   c. decontamination
   d. workplace safety ____

33. If the label on a disinfection product includes the word *concentrate*, it means that the product must be:
   a. used without water
   b. heated during use
   c. diluted before use
   d. heated before use ____

34. Quat solutions are _____ disinfectants when used properly in the salon.
   a. very effective
   b. somewhat effective
   c. never effective
   d. dangerous ____

35. Using _____ bleach can damage metal and plastic.
    a. too little
    b. diluted
    c. any amount of
    d. too much
    ____

36. Fumigants are _____ in salons because they produce potentially harmful formaldehyde gas.
    a. used carefully
    b. no longer used
    c. used after hours
    d. only used sometimes
    ____

37. Never let disinfectants such as phenols and quats come in contact with your:
    a. implements
    b. skin
    c. gloves
    d. clothing
    ____

38. Items that are _____ are also considered absorbent.
    a. phenolic
    b. parasitic
    c. pathogenic
    d. porous
    ____

39. Salons should keep a _____ that identifies each time a piece of equipment is used, cleaned, disinfected, tested, and maintained.
    a. list
    b. diary
    c. logbook
    d. journal
    ____

40. There is no additive, powder, or tablet that eliminates the need for you to _____ equipment such as whirlpool spas.
    a. clean and sterilize
    b. clean and disinfect
    c. clean and maintain
    d. clean and immunize
    ____

41. Not having _____ available poses a health risk to anyone exposed to hazardous materials and violates federal and state regulations.
    a. MSDSs
    b. MRSAs
    c. HRVs
    d. CDCs
    ____

42. Antimicrobial and antibacterial soaps are _____ regular soaps or detergents.
    a. slightly more effective than
    b. no more effective than
    c. just as effective as
    d. slightly less effective than
    ____

43. The _____ include hand washing, wearing gloves, and properly handling and disposing of items that may have been contaminated by blood or other body fluids.
    a. Universal Preconditions
    b. Universal Provisions
    c. Universal Precautions
    d. Universal Preparations ____

44. After they have been properly cleaned and disinfected, implements should be stored in a(n) _____ container.
    a. permanently sealed
    b. disposable
    c. clean, uncovered
    d. clean, covered ____

45. When cleaning and disinfecting a _____, remove the impeller, footplate, and any other removable parts according to the manufacturer's instructions.
    a. whirlpool foot spa
    b. air-jet basin
    c. pipe-less foot spa
    d. disinfecting foot spa ____

46. At the end of every day, you should properly clean the nonwhirlpool foot basin or tub and then add the appropriate amount of disinfectant and let it soak for:
    a. 10 minutes
    b. 5 minutes
    c. 1 minute
    d. 10 seconds ____

47. Before beginning any service, you should wash your hands using pump soap, water, and a:
    a. chemical disinfectant
    b. clean, disinfected nail brush
    c. clean, disinfected sponge
    d. chemical exfoliant ____

48. Something caused by or capable of being transmitted by infection is called:
    a. infectious
    b. contagious
    c. diseased
    d. fungicidal ____

49. The one-celled microorganisms having both plant and animal characteristics are called:
    a. flagella
    b. fungi
    c. cocci
    d. bacteria ____

50. The transmission of blood or body fluids through touching, kissing, coughing, sneezing, or talking is known as _____ transmission.
    a. sanitary
    b. infection
    c. sterile
    d. direct ____

51. Transmission of blood or body fluids through contact with a(n) _____, such as a razor or an environmental surface, is indirect transmission.
    a. disinfected contaminated object
    b. local contaminated object
    c. intermediate contaminated object
    d. unidentified flying object ____

52. Various poisonous substances produced by some microorganisms are called:
    a. tinea
    b. toxins
    c. bacteria
    d. flagella ____

53. A disease that is spread by contact from one person to another person is a(n):
    a. contagious disease
    b. infectious disease
    c. occupational disease
    d. systemic disease ____

54. A disease caused by pathogenic microorganisms that enter the body, and which may or may not be spread from one person to another person, is a(n):
    a. systemic disease
    b. infectious disease
    c. occupational disease
    d. contagious disease ____

55. The scientific name for plantar warts is:
    a. human immunodeficiency virus (HIV)
    b. human papilloma virus (HPV)
    c. acquired immune deficiency syndrome (AIDS)
    d. hepatitis B virus (HBV) ____

56. Any organism of microscopic to submicroscopic size is a(n):
    a. staphylococci
    b. streptococci
    c. mycobacterium
    d. microorganism ____

57. The removal of potentially infectious materials on an item's surface and the removal of visible debris or residue is called:
    a. disinfection
    b. cleaning
    c. decontamination
    d. sterilization ____

58. A(n) _____ disease affects the body as a whole, often due to under- or over-functioning of internal glands or organs.
    a. systemic
    b. infectious
    c. occupational
    d. contagious ____

59. The determination of the nature of a disease from its
    symptoms and/or tests is a(n):
    **a.** analysis               **c.** direct transmission
    **b.** disinfection        **d.** diagnosis      ____

60. A(n) _____ is a condition in which the body reacts
    to injury, irritation, or infection.
    **a.** allergy              **c.** contamination
    **b.** inflammation      **d.** exposure incident      ____

61. A parasitic disease is caused by:
    **a.** bacteria             **c.** parasites
    **b.** bacilli              **d.** cocci      ____

62. A(n) _____ is a submicroscopic particle that
    infects and resides in cells of biological organisms and is
    capable of replication only through taking over the host
    cell's reproductive function.
    **a.** cocci               **c.** bacterium
    **b.** virus               **d.** parasite      ____

63. The virus that causes AIDS is:
    **a.** hepatitis B virus (HBV)
    **b.** human papilloma virus (HPV)
    **c.** hepatitis C virus (HCV)
    **d.** human immunodeficiency virus (HIV)      ____

64. Contact with nonintact skin, blood, body fluid, or other
    potentially infectious materials that is the result of the
    performance of an employee's duties is a(n):
    **a.** allergy              **c.** contamination
    **b.** inflammation      **d.** exposure incident      ____

65. The scientific name for barber's itch is:
    **a.** tinea capitis        **c.** tinea barbae
    **b.** tinea pedis          **d.** tinea spirilla      ____

66. Organisms that grow, feed, and find shelter on or in another
    organism, while contributing nothing to the survival of that
    organism, are:
    **a.** cocci               **c.** parasites
    **b.** bacilli             **d.** lawyers      ____

67. The presence, or the reasonably anticipated presence, of potentially infectious materials on an item's surface or visible debris or residues is called:
   a. infection
   b. contamination
   c. inflammation
   d. allergy
   ____

68. The term _____ describes a ringworm fungus of the foot.
   a. tinea capitis
   b. tinea spirilla
   c. tinea barbae
   d. tinea pedis
   ____

69. A reaction due to extreme sensitivity to certain foods, chemicals, or other normally harmless substances is a(n):
   a. allergy
   b. contamination
   c. inflammation
   d. infection
   ____

70. A(n) _____ is produced by organisms, including bacteria, viruses, fungi, and parasites.
   a. systemic disease
   b. infectious disease
   c. pathogenic disease
   d. contagious disease
   ____

71. Illnesses resulting from conditions associated with employment are:
   a. contagious diseases
   b. occupational diseases
   c. pathogenic diseases
   d. systemic diseases
   ____

72. A(n) _____ is an abnormal condition of all or part of the body, or its systems or organs, that makes the body incapable of functioning normally.
   a. allergy
   b. infection
   c. disease
   d. contamination
   ____

# 6 General Anatomy and Physiology

## MULTIPLE CHOICE

1. The basic unit of all living things is the:
   a. anatomy
   b. cell
   c. muscle
   d. nerve ____

2. The dense active protoplasm found in the center of the cell is:
   a. cytoplasm
   b. cell membrane
   c. nucleus
   d. chromatid ____

3. Human cells reproduce by mitosis, dividing into two identical cells called:
   a. mother cells
   b. daughter cells
   c. father cells
   d. son cells ____

4. The _____ is the protoplasm of a cell except for the protoplasm in the nucleus.
   a. cystine
   b. neuron
   c. cytoplasm
   d. mandible ____

5. The chemical process through which cells are nourished and carry out their activities is called:
   a. metabolism
   b. mitosis
   c. meiosis
   d. respiration ____

6. The constructive phase of metabolism is called:
   a. anabolism
   b. catabolism
   c. mitosis
   d. meiosis ____

7. Which type of tissue contracts and moves various parts of the body?
   a. nerve tissue
   b. muscle tissue
   c. connective tissue
   d. epithelial tissue ____

8. Which type of tissue lines the heart and the digestive and respiratory organs?
   a. nerve tissue
   b. muscle tissue
   c. connective tissue
   d. epithelial tissue ____

9. The connection between two or more bones is called a:
   a. ligament
   b. joint
   c. tendon
   d. muscle ____

10. The _____ is the larger of the two bones that form the leg below the knee.
    a. patella
    b. fibula
    c. tibia
    d. femur
    ____

11. The oval, bony case that protects the brain is the:
    a. cranium
    b. facial skeleton
    c. hyoid bone
    d. thorax
    ____

12. The maxillae bones form the:
    a. lower jaw
    b. upper jaw
    c. upper arm
    d. forearm
    ____

13. The two bones that form the sides and crown (top) of the cranium are the:
    a. parietal bones
    b. occipital bones
    c. lacrimal bones
    d. zygomatic bones
    ____

14. The inner and larger bone in the forearm, attached to the wrist and located on the side of the little finger is the:
    a. carpus
    b. ulna
    c. metacarpus
    d. radius
    ____

15. The foot is made up of _____ bones.
    a. 6
    b. 11
    c. 18
    d. 26
    ____

16. Which muscles are also known as the smooth muscles?
    a. nonstriated muscles
    b. cardiac muscles
    c. striated muscles
    d. trapezius muscles
    ____

17. The part of the muscle that does not move is the:
    a. belly
    b. insertion
    c. origin
    d. tendon
    ____

18. The broad muscle that covers the top of the head is the:
    a. temporal
    b. epicranius
    c. deltoid
    d. occipital
    ____

19. The _____ are the muscles that straighten the wrist, hand, and fingers to form a straight line.
    a. extensors
    b. pronators
    c. supinators
    d. flexors
    ____

20. The muscles at the base of the fingers that draw the fingers together are the:
    a. flexors
    c. extensors
    b. abductors
    d. adductors ____

21. The system of nerves that carries impulses or messages to and from the central nervous system is called the:
    a. involuntary nervous system
    c. autonomic nerve system
    b. voluntary nervous system
    d. peripheral nervous system ____

22. Sensory nerve endings called _____ are located close to the surface of the skin.
    a. reactors
    c. capillaries
    b. receptors
    d. aural neurons ____

23. The largest artery in the human body is the:
    a. jugular
    c. aorta
    b. ventricle
    d. carotid ____

24. The main blood supply of the arms and hands are the:
    a. facial and superficial arteries
    b. ulnar and radial arteries
    c. radial and posterior arteries
    d. ulnar and external jugular arteries ____

25. The popliteal artery supplies blood to the foot and divides into two separate arteries known as the:
    a. anterior tibial and posterior tibial arteries
    b. anterior tibial and dorsalis pedis arteries
    c. internal and external jugular arteries
    d. supraorbital and infraorbital arteries ____

26. The _____ is the primary nasal muscle of concern to cosmetologists.
    a. platysmua
    c. popliteal
    b. procerus
    d. pronator ____

27. The mental nerve affects the skin of the:
    a. lower eyelid, side of the nose, upper lip, and mouth
    b. nose
    c. forehead, scalp, eyebrow, and upper eyelid
    d. lower lip and chin ____

28. The _____ cranial nerve is the chief motor nerve of the face.
    a. fourth
    b. fifth
    c. sixth
    d. seventh          ____

29. The greater occipital nerve is located at the _____ of the head and affects the scalp as far up as the top of the head.
    a. top
    b. back
    c. left side
    d. right side          ____

30. The median nerve supplies impulses to the:
    a. fingers
    b. wrist
    c. arm and hand
    d. arm and wrist          ____

31. The deep peroneal nerve is located in the:
    a. front of the arm
    b. front of the leg
    c. back of the leg
    d. front of the leg          ____

32. Valves are structures that temporarily close a passage or permit blood flow in:
    a. all directions
    b. only two directions
    c. only one direction
    d. only three directions          ____

33. Deoxygenated blood flows from the body into the:
    a. left atrium
    b. right atrium
    c. left ventricle
    d. right ventricle          ____

34. White blood cells are also known as:
    a. leukocytes
    b. hemoglobins
    c. platelets
    d. capillaries          ____

35. Blood _____ the body's temperature.
    a. has no effect upon
    b. plays a role in equalizing
    c. is the only factor affecting
    d. is only capable of raising          ____

36. The _____ supplies blood to the muscles of the eye.
    a. inferior labial artery
    b. infraorbital nerve
    c. infraorbital artery
    d. intratrochlear nerve          ____

37. The _____ drain(s) the tissue spaces of excess interstitial fluid.
    a. capillaries
    b. lymphatic system
    c. lymph nodes
    d. middle temporal artery ____

38. The _____ is a gland of the endocrine system that secretes enzyme-producing cells that are responsible for digesting carbohydrates, proteins, and fats.
    a. spleen
    b. thyroid
    c. lymph node
    d. pancreas ____

39. The _____ glands secrete about 30 steroid hormones and control metabolic processes of the body, including the fight-or-flight response.
    a. exocrine
    b. adrenal
    c. endocrine
    d. pituitary ____

40. Digestive _____ are chemicals that change certain types of food into a soluble form that can be used by the body.
    a. exocrines
    b. endocrines
    c. enzymes
    d. platelets ____

41. The organ that controls the body is the:
    a. heart
    b. brain
    c. stomach
    d. liver ____

42. The organs that control the body's vision are the:
    a. kidneys
    b. lungs
    c. intestines
    d. eyes ____

43. The heart is the organ that circulates the body's:
    a. lymph
    b. blood
    c. water
    d. spinal fluid ____

44. The organs that excretes water and waste products are the:
    a. intestines
    b. lungs
    c. kidneys
    d. eyes ____

45. The lungs supply _____ to the blood.
    a. hydrogen
    b. nitrogen
    c. oxygen
    d. carbon dioxide ____

46. The _____ is the organ that removes waste created by digestion.
    a. stomach
    c. intestine
    b. liver
    d. kidney                              ____

47. The _____ covers the body and is the external protective coating.
    a. scapula
    c. skin
    b. blood
    d. exoskeleton                         ____

48. The _____ are the organs that digest food.
    a. intestines and kidneys
    c. intestines and stomach
    b. intestines and liver
    d. kidneys and stomach                 ____

49. The _____ system controls the steady movement of the blood through the body.
    a. integumentary
    c. respiratory
    b. circulatory
    d. lymphatic                           ____

50. The _____ system changes food into nutrients and wastes.
    a. lymphatic
    c. integumentary
    b. endocrine
    d. digestive                           ____

51. The _____ system affects the growth, development, sexual functions, and health of the entire body.
    a. endocrine
    c. digestive
    b. excretory
    d. reproductive                        ____

52. The _____ system purifies the body by the elimination of waste matter.
    a. endocrine
    c. digestive
    b. excretory
    d. reproductive                        ____

53. The _____ system serves as a protective coating and helps regulate the body's temperature.
    a. lymphatic
    c. skeletal
    b. integumentary
    d. nervous                             ____

54. The _____ system protects the body from disease by developing immunities and destroying disease-causing toxins and bacteria.
    a. skeletal
    c. endocrine
    b. respiratory
    d. lymphatic                           ____

55. The _____ system covers, shapes, and supports the skeleton tissue.
    a. skeletal
    b. muscular
    c. nervous
    d. integumentary
    ____

56. The _____ system controls and coordinates all other systems inside and outside of the body and makes them work harmoniously and efficiently.
    a. lymphatic
    b. endocrine
    c. integumentary
    d. nervous
    ____

57. The _____ system controls the processes by which plants and animals produce offspring.
    a. reproductive
    b. genetic
    c. hereditary
    d. familial
    ____

58. The _____ system enables breathing, supplying the body with oxygen and eliminating carbon dioxide as a waste product.
    a. nervous
    b. reproductive
    c. respiratory
    d. endocrine
    ____

59. The _____ system forms the physical foundation of the body.
    a. skeletal
    b. muscular
    c. nervous
    d. reproductive
    ____

60. The study of the human body structures that can be seen with the naked eye and how the body parts are organized is:
    a. physiology
    b. histology
    c. myology
    d. anatomy
    ____

61. Physiology is the study of the functions and activities performed by the:
    a. body's elements
    b. body's structures
    c. body's shapes
    d. body's muscles
    ____

62. The study of tiny structures found in living tissues is known as histology or:
    a. microanatomy
    b. microscopic physiology
    c. microscopic anatomy
    d. microphysiology
    ____

63. Neurology is the study of the structure, function, and pathology of the:
    a. muscular system
    b. integumentary system
    c. skeletal system
    d. nervous system
    ____

**64.** The study of the nature, structure, function, and diseases of the muscles is:

    **a.** anatomy                  **c.** histology

    **b.** myology                **d.** physiology     ____

**65.** Osteology is the study of the anatomy, structure, and function of the:

    **a.** bones                   **c.** muscles

    **b.** nerves                  **d.** skin     ____

# CHAPTER 7

# Skin Structure, Growth, and Nutrition

## MULTIPLE CHOICE

1. A(n) _____ is a physician who specializes in diseases and disorders of the skin, hair, and nails.
   - **a.** histologist
   - **b.** dermatologist
   - **c.** esthetician
   - **d.** pediatrician
   ____

2. Healthy skin is:
   - **a.** smooth with a fine-grained texture
   - **b.** highly acidic
   - **c.** dry and tough
   - **d.** inflexible
   ____

3. All of the following are appendages of the skin *except*:
   - **a.** sudoriferous glands
   - **b.** nails
   - **c.** adrenal glands
   - **d.** hair
   ____

4. Which of the following correctly identifies the layers of skin and fat from the outermost layer to the innermost layer?
   - **a.** dermis, subcutaneous, epidermis
   - **b.** epidermis, subcutaneous, dermis
   - **c.** dermis, epidermis, subcutaneous
   - **d.** epidermis, dermis, subcutaneous
   ____

5. Cells that are almost dead and pushed to the surface to replace cells are shed from the:
   - **a.** stratum corneum
   - **b.** stratum lucidum
   - **c.** stratum germinativum
   - **d.** stratum granulosum
   ____

6. The layer directly beneath the epidermis is the:
   - **a.** reticular layer
   - **b.** stratum spinosum
   - **c.** papillary layer
   - **d.** subcutaneous tissue
   ____

7. Which type of tissue gives smoothness and contour to the body and provides a protective cushion?
   - **a.** subcutaneous tissue
   - **b.** cardiac tissue
   - **c.** muscle tissue
   - **d.** nerve tissue
   ____

8. Which nerve fibers are distributed to the arrector pili muscles attached to the hair follicles?
   - **a.** motor nerve fibers
   - **b.** sensory nerve fibers
   - **c.** secretory nerve fibers
   - **d.** impulse nerve fibers
   ____

9. Nerves that regulate the secretion of perspiration and sebum are:
   a. motor nerve fibers
   b. sensory nerve fibers
   c. secretory nerve fibers
   d. impulse nerve fibers _____

10. Basic sensations such as touch, pain, heat, cold, and pressure are registered by:
    a. arrector pili muscles
    b. nerve endings
    c. sweat pores
    d. hair follicles _____

11. The amount and type of pigment produced by an individual is determined primarily by his or her:
    a. genes
    b. gender
    c. sun exposure
    d. age _____

12. Skin gets its strength, form, and flexibility from:
    a. collagen and keratin
    b. sebum and melanin
    c. keratin and elastin
    d. collagen and elastin _____

13. The sudoriferous glands do *not*:
    a. help the body regulate temperature
    b. eliminate waste products
    c. secrete a lubricating substance
    d. exist on the palms or soles _____

14. To keep your body healthy, you must be sure that what you eat:
    a. prevents hydration
    b. causes fatigue
    c. has a pleasant taste
    d. regulates the function of your cells _____

15. Which vitamin accelerates the skin's healing processing and is vitally important in fighting the aging process?
    a. vitamin A
    b. vitamin C
    c. vitamin D
    d. vitamin E _____

16. The epidermis is the _____ layer of the skin.
    a. healthiest
    b. thickest
    c. thinnest
    d. most important _____

17. The scalp has larger and deeper _____ than the skin on the rest of the body.
    a. melanocytes
    b. Propionibacterium acnes
    c. sensory nerve fibers
    d. hair follicles _____

18. It is _____ for a cosmetologist to completely remove a client's callus in the salon.
    a. safe
    b. legal
    c. prohibited
    d. recommended _____

19. One of the best ways to follow a healthy diet is to read:
    a. magazine articles
    b. food labels
    c. diet books
    d. legal guidelines _____

20. Emotional stress and hormone imbalances can increase the flow of:
    a. sebum
    b. spinal fluid
    c. lymph
    d. pus _____

21. To function correctly, the body needs:
    a. carbohydrates, proteins, and vitamins
    b. carbohydrates, proteins, vitamins, and fats
    c. carbohydrates, fats, proteins, vitamins, and minterals
    d. carbohydrates, fats, proteins, vitamins, minerals, and water _____

22. The USDA recommends that people eat:
    a. zero salt and zero sugar
    b. large amounts of salt and sugar
    c. moderate amounts of salt and sugar
    d. moderate amounts of salt and no sugar _____

23. Vitamin pills are considered:
    a. nutritional requirements
    b. nutritional supplements
    c. cosmetics
    d. prescription medications _____

24. The appropriate amount of water that a person should drink each day is determined by the person's:
    a. weight
    b. age
    c. skin color
    d. medical history _____

25. Lack of water is the principal cause of:
    a. daytime fatigue
    b. daytime hunger
    c. daytime mood swings
    d. daytime memory loss _____

26. Small, cone-shaped elevations at the bottom of the hair follicles are:
    a. melanocytes
    b. papules
    c. dermal papillae
    d. secretory coils _____

27. The layer of the epidermis where the process of skin cell shedding begins is the:
    a. stratum corneum
    b. stratum lucidum
    c. stratum germinativum
    d. stratum spinosum          ____

28. The coiled base of the sudoriferous gland is known as the:
    a. secretory coil
    b. sweat duct
    c. sebaceous gland
    d. elastin coil          ____

29. A small, round elevation on the skin that contains no fluid but may develop pus is a:
    a. comedo
    b. papule
    c. callus
    d. pustule          ____

30. Fatty tissue found below the dermis is _____ tissue.
    a. secretory
    b. sudoriferous
    c. subcutaneous
    d. sensory          ____

31. An inflamed pimple containing pus is a:
    a. papillary
    b. pustule
    c. callus
    d. comedo          ____

32. The outer layer of the epidermis is the _____ layer.
    a. papillary
    b. reticular
    c. tactile
    d. epidermal          ____

33. The layer of the epidermis that is composed of cells filled with keratin is the:
    a. stratum spinosum
    b. stratum granulosum
    c. stratum germinativum
    d. stratum corneum          ____

34. A fatty or oily secretion that lubricates the skin and preserves the softness of the hair is:
    a. sebum
    b. lymph
    c. pus
    d. melanin          ____

35. The layer of the epidermis also known as the basal cell layer is the:
    a. stratum lucidum
    b. stratum spinosum
    c. stratum corneum
    d. stratum germinativum          ____

# 8 Skin Disorders and Diseases

## MULTIPLE CHOICE

1. Approximately _____ percent of skin aging is caused by the rays of the sun.
   a. 50 to 55 percent
   c. 70 to 75 percent
   b. 60 to 65 percent
   d. 80 to 85 percent    ____

2. It is recommended that you wear a broad-spectrum sunscreen with an SPF of at least _____ on a daily basis.
   a. 5
   c. 15
   b. 8
   d. 30    ____

3. A _____ is an abnormal rounded solid lump larger than a papule and located above, within, or under the skin.
   a. tubercle
   c. macula
   b. mole
   d. bulla    ____

4. Which of these terms refers to thin dry or oily plates of epidermal flakes?
   a. fissures
   c. pustules
   b. crust
   d. scales    ____

5. Keratin-filled cysts that appear just under the epidermis and have no visible openings are:
   a. milia
   c. crust
   b. ulcers
   d. pustules    ____

6. An open comedo is commonly known as a:
   a. mole
   c. blackhead
   b. birthmark
   d. whitehead    ____

7. Which of these is an uncomfortable, and often chronic, disease of the skin, characterized by inflammation, scaling, and sometimes severe itching?
   a. eczema
   c. psoriasis
   b. acne
   d. herpes simplex    ____

8. A _____ is an abnormal brown or wine-colored skin discoloration with a circular and irregular shape.
   a. mole
   c. chloasma
   b. stain
   d. lentigo    ____

9. The absence of melanin pigment from the body and skin sensitivity to light are signs of:
   a. nevus
   b. lentignes
   c. asteatosis
   d. albinism ____

10. What is the most dangerous type of skin cancer, often characterized by black or dark brown patches on the skin that may appear uneven in texture, jagged, or raised?
    a. basal cell carcinoma
    b. malignant melanoma
    c. squamous cell melanoma
    d. verruca cell ____

11. A cosmetologist must not serve a client who is suffering from an inflamed skin disorder, regardless of whether it is infectious, unless the client:
    a. needs a facial quickly for an important event such as a wedding
    b. declares that he or she is practicing doctor-prescribed home care
    c. has a physician's note permitting the client to receive services
    d. signs a waiver clearing the cosmetologist and the salon of liability ____

12. A skin condition caused by inflammation of the sebaceous glands is:
    a. contact dermatitis
    b. irritant contact dermatitis
    c. allergic contact dermatitis
    d. seborrheic dermatitis ____

13. The term _____ refers to an abnormal coloration that accompanies a skin disorder or systemic disorder.
    a. anhidrosis
    b. bromhidrosis
    c. dyschromia
    d. conjunctivitis ____

14. A(n) _____ is a type of keratoma.
    a. callus
    b. keloid
    c. lesion
    d. excoriation ____

15. Acne is a skin disorder characterized by chronic inflammation of the _____ gland.
    a. sudoriferous
    b. sebaceous
    c. sweat
    d. adrenaline ____

16. Acne is affected by both genetic and _____ factors.
    a. anaerobic
    b. malignant
    c. noncomedogenic
    d. hormonal
    ____

17. Noncomedogenic products are specifically designed not to clog the:
    a. bullas
    b. dyschromias
    c. follicles
    d. free radicals
    ____

18. People have _____ over the extrinsic factors that affect aging, but not the intrinsic factors.
    a. no control
    b. very little control
    c. considerable control
    d. total control
    ____

19. The best defense against pollutants is to:
    a. wear sunscreen whenever you are outside
    b. avoid touching your face with your hands
    c. follow a good daily skin care routine
    d. wear long-sleeved clothing when you are outdoors
    ____

20. Irritant contact dermatitis occurs when irritating substances temporarily damage the:
    a. dermis
    b. epidermis
    c. papillary layer
    d. hair follicles
    ____

21. A pustule is a raised, inflamed pimple containing _____ in the top of the lesion.
    a. water
    b. blood
    c. lymph
    d. pus
    ____

22. A _____ is a large, protruding, pocket-like lesion filled with sebum.
    a. closed comedo
    b. sebaceous cyst
    c. bulla
    d. miliaria rubra
    ____

23. Any flat spot or discoloration on the skin left after a pimple has healed is a:
    a. macule
    b. leukoderma
    c. milia
    d. scale
    ____

24. Foul-smelling perspiration caused by bacteria is:
    a. hyperhidrosis
    b. miliaria rubra
    c. anhidrosis
    d. bromhidrosis
    ____

**25.** A(n) _____ is a slightly raised mark on the skin formed after an injury or lesion of the skin has healed.
   **a.** mole            **c.** scale
   **b.** scar            **d.** stain      ____

**26.** The contagious bacterial skin infection characterized by weeping lesions is:
   **a.** impetigo        **c.** eczema
   **b.** conjunctivitis    **d.** herpes simplex      ____

**27.** A _____ is an itchy, swollen lesion that lasts only a few hours.
   **a.** wheal         **c.** verruca
   **b.** vesicle        **d.** tubercle      ____

**28.** A(n) _____ is a crack in the skin that penetrates the dermis.
   **a.** ulcer         **c.** excoriation
   **b.** fissure       **d.** crust      ____

**29.** A small blister or sac containing clear fluid, lying within or just beneath the epidermis is a:
   **a.** tubercle      **c.** vesicle
   **b.** tumor        **d.** wheal      ____

**30.** The acute inflammatory disorder of the sweat glands, characterized by the eruption of small red vesicles and accompanied by burning, itching skin is:
   **a.** hyperhidrosis    **c.** anhidrosis
   **b.** miliaria rubra    **d.** bromhidrosia      ____

# CHAPTER 9 Nail Structure and Growth

## MULTIPLE CHOICE

1. A normal, healthy nail:
   - **a.** is completely inflexible
   - **b.** has a spotted surface
   - **c.** is shiny
   - **d.** is white and opaque        ____

2. The portion of the living skin on which the nail plate sits is called the:
   - **a.** nail bed
   - **b.** cuticle
   - **c.** matrix
   - **d.** ligament        ____

3. The _____ is the whitish, half-moon shape at the base of the nail.
   - **a.** sidewall
   - **b.** lunula
   - **c.** root
   - **d.** free edge        ____

4. The part of the nail plate that extends over the tip of the finger or toe is the:
   - **a.** free edge
   - **b.** matrix
   - **c.** bed epithelium
   - **d.** sidewall        ____

5. A _____ is a tough band of fibrous tissue that connects bones or holds an organ in place.
   - **a.** muscle
   - **b.** ligament
   - **c.** tendon
   - **d.** nerve        ____

6. The _____ is the fold of skin overlapping the side of the nail.
   - **a.** eponychium
   - **b.** hyponychium
   - **c.** nail groove
   - **d.** sidewall        ____

7. After an injury, infection, or disease, the natural nail will return to its healthy growth as long as the _____ is healthy and undamaged.
   - **a.** lateral nail fold
   - **b.** lunula
   - **c.** matrix
   - **d.** nail plate        ____

8. Replacement of the natural fingernail usually takes about:
   - **a.** 6 to 12 months
   - **b.** 4 to 6 months
   - **c.** 4 to 8 weeks
   - **d.** 2 to 8 months        ____

9. The finger nail on the _____ typically grows slowest.
   a. thumb
   c. pinkie finger
   b. middle finger
   d. index finger    ____

10. The nail has a water content between:
    a. 10 and 15 percent
    c. 20 and 45 percent
    b. 1 and 5 percent
    d. 15 and 25 percent    ____

11. The natural nail is an appendage of the:
    a. dermis
    c. skin
    b. epidermis
    d. skeleton    ____

12. The appearance of the nails can reflect the general health of the:
    a. body
    c. muscular system
    b. skin
    d. skeletal system    ____

13. The _____ is relatively porous and will allow water to pass through.
    a. nail bed
    c. nail plate
    b. matrix
    d. eponychium    ____

14. The matrix contains:
    a. lymph and blood vessels
    b. nerves, lymph, and blood vessels
    c. water and blood vessels
    d. water, lymph, and blood vessels    ____

15. Tissue that adheres directly to the natural nail plate but which can be easily removed with gentle scraping is:
    a. ligament
    c. eponychium
    b. hyponychium
    d. cuticle    ____

16. Cosmetologists are allowed to _____ the eponychium.
    a. cut
    c. push back
    b. trim
    d. file    ____

17. Cuticle moisturizers, softeners, and conditioners are *not* designed to treat the:
    a. cuticle
    c. sidewalls
    b. nail plate
    d. hyponychium    ____

**18.** Toenails are thicker and harder than fingernails because the _____ of the toenail is longer than that of the fingernail.

    **a.** nail bed           **c.** lunula

    **b.** matrix             **d.** eponychium    ____

**19.** Unlike healthy hair, healthy nails are not _____ periodically.

    **a.** cut                **c.** shed

    **b.** cleaned          **d.** maintained    ____

**20.** It takes about _____ for toenails to be fully replaced.

    **a.** three to six months

    **b.** six to nine months

    **c.** nine months to one year

    **d.** one year to fifteen months    ____

**21.** The living skin at the base of the natural nail plate that covers the matrix area is the:

    **a.** eponychium       **c.** cuticle

    **b.** hyponychium     **d.** lunula    ____

**22.** The thin layer of tissue between the nail plate and the nail bed is the:

    **a.** bed eponychium     **c.** lateral nail fold

    **b.** bed epithelium      **d.** onyx    ____

**23.** The slightly thickened layer of skin that lies between the fingertip and free edge of the natural nail plate is the:

    **a.** epithelium        **c.** sidewall

    **b.** eponychium       **d.** hyponychium    ____

**24.** The dead, colorless tissue attached to the natural nail plate is known as the:

    **a.** nail bed          **c.** nail groove

    **b.** nail fold         **d.** nail cuticle    ____

**25.** The _____ is the area where the nail plate cells are formed.

    **a.** cuticle           **c.** matrix

    **b.** lunula           **d.** free edge    ____

# CHAPTER 10 Nail Disorders and Diseases

## MULTIPLE CHOICE

1. A normal healthy nail is firm and flexible and should be:
   - **a.** smooth and unspotted
   - **b.** uneven and unspotted
   - **c.** long and unspotted
   - **d.** short and unspotted _____

2. If a client has ridges running vertically down the length of the natural nail plate, it is recommended that you:
   - **a.** file them aggressively
   - **b.** buff them carefully
   - **c.** thin the nail plate
   - **d.** refer the client to a physician _____

3. The medical term for fungal infections associated with the feet is:
   - **a.** tinea pathogenic
   - **b.** tinea pedis
   - **c.** tinea alopecia
   - **d.** paronychia _____

4. A typical bacterial infection on the nail plate can be identified in the early stages as a _____ spot that becomes darker in its advanced stages.
   - **a.** orange-red
   - **b.** white-gray
   - **c.** blue-green
   - **d.** yellow-green _____

5. The separation and falling off of a nail from the nail bed is a sign of:
   - **a.** onychia
   - **b.** paronychia
   - **c.** onychomadesis
   - **d.** pyogenic granuloma _____

6. Which of the following does *not* cause onychorrhexis?
   - **a.** injury to the matrix
   - **b.** heredity
   - **c.** aggressive filing techniques
   - **d.** insufficient use of cuticle removers _____

7. Tiny pits or severe roughness on the surface of the nail are signs of which condition?
   - **a.** paronychia
   - **b.** onychocryptosis
   - **c.** nail psoriasis
   - **d.** onychomycosis _____

8. The term _____ refers to a condition caused by injury or disease of the nail unit.
   - **a.** nail psoriasis
   - **b.** nail pterygium
   - **c.** nail disorder
   - **d.** nail service _____

9. Splinter hemorrhages are caused by physical trauma or injury to the:
   a. nail plate
   b. nail bed
   c. free edge
   d. lunula
   ____

10. Nail fungi can be transmitted through _____ instruments.
    a. sterilized
    b. disinfected
    c. contaminated
    d. disposable
    ____

11. Onychomadesis can affect:
    a. only fingernails
    b. only toenails
    c. neither fingernails nor toenails
    d. both fingernails and toenails
    ____

12. A cosmetologist can disobey state or federal rules and regulations:
    a. if the client signs a waiver
    b. under no circumstances
    c. with the client's verbal permission
    d. if the salon owner gives permission
    ____

13. Which condition is characterized by nails that are noticeably thin, flexible, and white?
    a. melanonychia
    b. plicatured nail
    c. agnail
    d. eggshell nails
    ____

14. Which of the following is *not* a common cause of surface stains on nails?
    a. nail polish
    b. food dyes
    c. smoking
    d. poor blood circulation
    ____

15. The condition in which a blood clot forms under the nail plate, causing a dark purplish spot, is:
    a. discolored nails
    b. bruised nails
    c. eggshell nails
    d. plicatured nails
    ____

16. The condition in which the living skin around the nail splits and tears is:
    a. hangnail
    b. Beau's lines
    c. melanonychia
    d. onychophagy
    ____

17. The lifting of the nail plate from the bed without shedding is:
    a. onychosis
    b. onychocryptosis
    c. onycholysis
    d. onychomadesis        ____

18. The term _____ refers to significant darkening of the fingernails or toenails.
    a. melanonychia
    b. nail pterygium
    c. paronychia
    d. splinter hemorrhages        ____

19. A sharp bend in one corner of the nail plate creating increased curvature is symptomatic of:
    a. pincer nails
    b. bruised nails
    c. eggshell nails
    d. plicatured nails        ____

20. Depressions running across the width of the nail plate are:
    a. ridges
    b. splinters
    c. Beau's lines
    d. agnail        ____

## MULTIPLE CHOICE

1. The scientific study of hair, its diseases, and care is called:
   - **a.** dermatology
   - **b.** trichology
   - **c.** biology
   - **d.** cosmetology          ____

2. The two parts of a mature strand of human hair are the:
   - **a.** dermis and epidermis
   - **b.** hair shaft and hair follicle
   - **c.** hair shaft and hair root
   - **d.** hair root and hair follicle    ____

3. The tube-like depression or pocket in the skin or scalp that contains the hair root is the:
   - **a.** follicle
   - **b.** shaft
   - **c.** bulb
   - **d.** scalp          ____

4. Hair follicles are *not* found on the:
   - **a.** forehead area
   - **b.** back of the hands
   - **c.** soles of the feet
   - **d.** back of the neck          ____

5. The _____ is a tiny, involuntary muscle in the base of the hair follicle.
   - **a.** medulla
   - **b.** arrector pili
   - **c.** tinea
   - **d.** dermal papilla          ____

6. An oily substance secreted from the sebaceous glands is:
   - **a.** sweat
   - **b.** lymph
   - **c.** catagen
   - **d.** sebum          ____

7. For chemicals to penetrate a healthy cuticle hair layer, they must have:
   - **a.** no pH
   - **b.** a neutral pH
   - **c.** an alkaline pH
   - **d.** an acidic pH          ____

8. The medulla is composed of _____ cells.
   - **a.** rod-shaped
   - **b.** round
   - **c.** spiral-shaped
   - **d.** rectangular          ____

9. The process whereby living cells mature and begin their journey up the hair shaft is:
   - **a.** anagen
   - **b.** catagen
   - **c.** keratinization
   - **d.** osmosis          ____

10. The five main elements that make up the chemical composition of human hair are carbon, oxygen, hydrogen, and:
    a. lead and zinc
    b. keratin and selenium
    c. boron and calcium
    d. nitrogen and sulfur ____

11. The chemical bonds that hold together the amino acid molecules are called:
    a. convex bonds
    b. peptide bonds
    c. helium bonds
    d. protein bonds ____

12. Which type of melanin provides natural colors ranging from red and ginger to yellow and blond tones?
    a. pheomelanin
    b. eumelanin
    c. polymelanin
    d. biomelanin ____

13. Asians tend to have:
    a. extremely straight hair
    b. extremely curly hair
    c. straight to wavy hair
    d. wavy to curly hair ____

14. To help minimize tangles in extremely curly hair when washing, you should use:
    a. a drying shampoo
    b. strong scalp manipulations
    c. a detangling rinse
    d. soap instead of shampoo ____

15. Hair texture is classified as:
    a. wavy, straight, or curly
    b. coarse, medium, or fine
    c. light, medium, or dark
    d. long, medium, or short ____

16. The measurement of individual hair strands on 1 square inch (2.5 square centimeters) of the scalp is:
    a. hair density
    b. hair elasticity
    c. hair texture
    d. hair porosity ____

17. Compared to hair with high porosity, chemical services performed on hair with low porosity require:
    a. neutral solutions
    b. more acidic solutions
    c. solutions of the same pH
    d. more alkaline solutions ____

18. Wet hair with normal elasticity will stretch up to _____ of its original length.
    a. 25 percent
    b. 40 percent
    c. 50 percent
    d. 70 percent ____

19. Oily scalp and hair can be treated by properly washing it:
    a. without shampoo
    b. with normalizing shampoo
    c. with conditioning shampoo
    d. with dry shampoo          ____

20. Which type of hair almost never has a medulla?
    a. oily
    b. pigmented
    c. dark
    d. vellus          ____

21. The growth phase during which new hair is produced is:
    a. patagen
    b. telogen
    c. anagen
    d. catagen          ____

22. The average growth of healthy scalp hair is:
    a. ½ inch (1.25 cm) per week
    b. 1 inch (2.5 cm) per week
    c. ½ inch (1.25 cm) per month
    d. 1 inch (2.5 cm) per month

23. The technical term used to describe gray hair is:
    a. canities
    b. tinea
    c. alopecia
    d. albino          ____

24. A condition of abnormal hair growth on areas of the body is:
    a. trichorrhexis
    b. ringed hair
    c. hypertrichosis
    d. electrolysis          ____

25. The medical term for dandruff is:
    a. canities
    b. pityriasis
    c. alopecia
    d. simplex          ____

26. The body can produce 11 of the 20 _____ that make up hair.
    a. amino acids
    b. COHNS elements
    c. disulfide bonds
    d. polypeptide chains          ____

27. Salt bonds account for about _____ of the hair's overall strength.
    a. one-quarter
    b. one-half
    c. one-third
    d. two-thirds          ____

28. The anagen phase generally lasts from three to five:
    a. days
    b. weeks
    c. months
    d. years          ____

29. Scalp hair grows _____ on women than on men.
    a. slower
    b. faster
    c. thinner
    d. thicker          ____

30. The _____ phase signals the end of the growth phase.
    a. cysteine
    b. cystine
    c. anagen
    d. catagen
    ____

31. Scalp massage _____ hair growth.
    a. increases
    b. decreases
    c. does not affect
    d. is necessary for
    ____

32. Compared to pigmented hair, gray hair is:
    a. neither coarser nor more resistant
    b. both coarser and more resistant
    c. coarser
    d. more resistant
    ____

33. Cross-sections of hair:
    a. are always round
    b. are always oval
    c. are always flattened oval
    d. can be almost any shape
    ____

34. Bald men are commonly perceived as:
    a. more assertive
    b. younger
    c. more physically attractive
    d. less successful
    ____

35. By age 35, almost _____ percent of both men and women show some degree of hair loss.
    a. 20
    b. 30
    c. 40
    d. 50
    ____

36. Finasteride is an oral prescription medication for hair loss that is meant for:
    a. men only
    b. women only
    c. men and women
    d. animals
    ____

37. Congenital canities manifests:
    a. at or before birth
    b. during adolescence
    c. during middle age
    d. in the later years of life
    ____

38. Dandruff can easily be mistaken for:
    a. tinea
    b. dry scalp
    c. pediculosis capitis
    d. trichoptilosis
    ____

**39.** Dandruff is believed to be caused by a:
- **a.** bacterium
- **b.** virus
- **c.** parasite
- **d.** fungus

_____

**40.** The most frequently encountered fungal infection resulting from hair services is:
- **a.** tinea barbae
- **b.** tinea capitis
- **c.** tinea pedis
- **d.** tinea favosa

_____

**41.** Tinea is characterized by:
- **a.** numbness
- **b.** blisters
- **c.** sudden hair loss
- **d.** itching

_____

**42.** The infestation of the hair and scalp with head lice is called:
- **a.** hypertrichosis
- **b.** trichoptilosis
- **c.** pediculosis capitis
- **d.** fragilitas crinium

_____

**43.** A carbuncle is similar to a furuncle, but is:
- **a.** smaller
- **b.** larger
- **c.** much darker in color
- **d.** much lighter in color

_____

**44.** Fine hair is _____ than coarse or medium hair.
- **a.** thicker
- **b.** harder to process
- **c.** less susceptible to damage from chemical services
- **d.** more fragile

_____

**45.** Coarse hair:
- **a.** has the smallest diameter of the three types of hair texture
- **b.** is the most common hair texture
- **c.** is not resistant to chemical services
- **d.** is stronger than fine hair

_____

**46.** The _____ is the outermost layer of hair.
- **a.** hair cuticle
- **b.** hair bulb
- **c.** hair follicle
- **d.** hair root

_____

**47.** The oil glands in the skin that are connected to the hair follicles are the _____ glands.
- **a.** systine
- **b.** simplex
- **c.** sebaceous
- **d.** scutulua

_____

**48.** A _____ bond is a physical bond easily broken by water or heat.

   **a.** hydrogen           **c.** hydrophobic

   **b.** hydrophillic         **d.** helix           ____

**49.** Hair is approximately _____ percent protein.

   **a.** 60               **c.** 80

   **b.** 70               **d.** 90           ____

**50.** Total scalp hair loss is known as:

   **a.** alopecia areata        **c.** alopecia totalis

   **b.** androgenetic alopecia    **d.** alopecia universalis   ____

**51.** Hypertrichosis is also known as:

   **a.** ringed hair         **c.** canities

   **b.** hirsuties           **d.** split ends       ____

**52.** The naturally occurring fungus that causes the symptoms of dandruff when it grows out of control is:

   **a.** medulla           **c.** malassezia

   **b.** monilethrix       **d.** hypertrichosis     ____

**53.** The _____ is the lowest part of a hair strand.

   **a.** hair root          **c.** hair cuticle

   **b.** hair bulb         **d.** hair follicle      ____

**54.** The technical term for beaded hair is:

   **a.** monilethrix       **c.** trichorrhexis nodosa

   **b.** fragilitas crinium    **d.** hypertrichosis     ____

**55.** A highly contagious skin disease caused by a parasite called a mite that burrows under the skin is:

   **a.** capitis            **c.** furuncle

   **b.** scabies           **d.** carbuncle      ____

**56.** The term for the spiral shape of a coiled protein is:

   **a.** matrix             **c.** helix

   **b.** cystine           **d.** cysteine       ____

**57.** Shaving, clipping, and cutting the hair on the head:

   **a.** makes it grow back faster

   **b.** makes it grow back darker

   **c.** makes it grow back coarser

   **d.** has no effect on hair growth                ____

58. Dry, sulfur-yellow, cup-like crusts on the scalp are called:
    a. tinea barbae
    c. scutula
    b. scabies
    d. wheals ____

59. The _____ are part of the integumentary system.
    a. hair, skin, and nails
    c. hair, glands, and nails
    b. hair, skin, nails, and glands
    d. nails, skin, and glands ____

60. The long, coarse, pigmented hair found on the scalp, legs, arms, and bodies of males and females is called _____.
    a. vellus hair
    c. extra hair
    b. lanugo hair
    d. terminal hair ____

61. The technical term for knotted hair is:
    a. trichorrhexis nodosa
    c. trichoptilosis
    b. monilethrix
    d. hypertrichosis ____

62. The _____ is the innermost layer of the hair.
    a. tinea
    c. medulla
    b. monilethrix
    d. scutula ____

63. Hair that forms in a circular pattern on the crown of the head is called:
    a. crown hair
    c. ringed hair
    b. cowlick
    d. whorl ____

64. The part of the hair located below the surface of the epidermis is the:
    a. hair root
    c. hair stream
    b. hair shaft
    d. hair bulb ____

65. A tuft of hair that stands straight up is a:
    a. cystine
    c. cortex
    b. cysteine
    d. cowlick ____

66. The ability of the hair to absorb moisture is called:
    a. hair absorbency
    c. hair saturation
    b. hair porosity
    d. hair stream ____

67. The middle layer of the hair is the:
    a. cortex
    c. canity
    b. carbuncle
    d. catagen ____

**68.** An autoimmune disorder that causes affected hair follicles to be mistakenly attacked by a person's own immune system is:

   **a.** androgenic alopecia       **c.** alopecia totalis

   **b.** alopecia areata           **d.** alopecia universalis    ____

**69.** Vellus hair is also known as:

   **a.** lanugo hair            **c.** malassezia hair

   **b.** lanthionine hair       **d.** monilethrix hair    ____

**70.** The medical term for ringworm is:

   **a.** tinea                **c.** tinea favosa

   **b.** tinea barbae          **d.** tinea capitis    ____

# CHAPTER 12 Basics of Chemistry

## MULTIPLE CHOICE

1. Inorganic chemistry is the study of substances that do not contain the element carbon, but may contain which element?
   - **a.** silicon
   - **b.** oxygen
   - **c.** hydrogen
   - **d.** nitrogen _____

2. A(n) _____ is a substance that cannot be broken down into simpler substances without loss of identity.
   - **a.** compound
   - **b.** ion
   - **c.** molecule
   - **d.** element _____

3. Chemically joining two or more atoms in definite proportions forms a(n):
   - **a.** acid
   - **b.** molecule
   - **c.** mixture
   - **d.** solvent _____

4. A(n) _____ is a stable physical mixture of two or more substances.
   - **a.** solution
   - **b.** emulsion
   - **c.** compound
   - **d.** element _____

5. A(n) _____ is a substance dissolved into a solution.
   - **a.** solvent
   - **b.** alkali
   - **c.** solute
   - **d.** acid _____

6. Liquids that are not capable of being mixed into stable solutions are considered:
   - **a.** emulsions
   - **b.** suspensions
   - **c.** miscible
   - **d.** immiscible _____

7. Solutions that contain undissolved particles that are visible to the naked eye are known as:
   - **a.** suspensions
   - **b.** mixtures
   - **c.** solutes
   - **d.** emulsions _____

8. A(n) _____ is a mixture of two or more immiscible substances united with the aid of a binder.
   - **a.** suspension
   - **b.** emulsion
   - **c.** mixture
   - **d.** solution _____

9. A(n) _____ is a substance that acts as a bridge to allow oil and water to mix or emulsify.
   a. reducing agent
   c. anion
   b. surfactant
   d. cation _____

10. The tail of a surfactant molecule is oil-loving or:
    a. miscible
    c. lipophilic
    b. immiscible
    d. hydrophilic _____

11. A molecule that carries an electric charge is called an:
    a. alkaline
    c. atom
    b. acid
    d. ion _____

12. Alpha hydroxy acids (AHAs):
    a. are used to exfoliate the skin
    c. are also known as bases
    b. feel slippery on the skin
    d. are used to soften the hair _____

13. An exothermic chemical reaction:
    a. produces a positive electrical charge
    b. produces a negative electrical charge
    c. absorbs heat
    d. releases heat _____

14. A substance that has a pH below 7.0 is considered to be:
    a. combustible
    c. acidic
    b. neutral
    d. alkaline _____

15. Alkanolamines are often used in place of ammonia because they:
    a. produce less odor
    c. have a better texture
    b. are much less expensive
    d. are much more effective _____

16. Which of these is *not* composed of organic chemicals?
    a. pesticides
    c. synthetic fabrics
    b. shampoos
    d. minerals _____

17. Elemental molecules contain two or more _____ of the same element in definite proportions.
    a. atoms
    c. cations
    b. ions
    d. silicones _____

18. Vapor is a(n) _____ that has evaporated into a gas-like state.
    a. element
    c. liquid
    b. solid
    d. chemical _____

**19.** An oxidizing agent is a substance that releases:
   **a.** hydrogen          **c.** oxygen
   **b.** nitrogen          **d.** carbon          ____

**20.** Pure substances:
   **a.** are united physically
   **b.** have unique chemical and physical properties
   **c.** can have any proportions
   **d.** are the same as physical mixtures          ____

**21.** Calamine lotion is an example of a(n):
   **a.** emulsion          **c.** solution
   **b.** mixture           **d.** suspension          ____

**22.** Water-in-oil emulsions feel _____ than oil-in-water emulsions.
   **a.** greasier          **c.** wetter
   **b.** hotter            **d.** colder          ____

**23.** A common use of _____ is raising the pH in hair products to allow the solution to penetrate the hair shaft.
   **a.** amino acid        **c.** alkaline solution
   **b.** ammonia           **d.** alpha hydroxy acids          ____

**24.** Volatile organic compounds contain _____ and evaporate very easily.
   **a.** carbon            **c.** oxygen
   **b.** hydrogen          **d.** nitrogen          ____

**25.** Which of these types of products has no pH?
   **a.** haircolor         **c.** shampoos
   **b.** relaxers          **d.** oils          ____

**26.** The chemical reaction that combines a substance with oxygen to produce an oxide is:
   **a.** combustion        **c.** ionization
   **b.** oxidization       **d.** reduction          ____

**27.** The term logarithm means multiples of:
   **a.** 5                 **c.** 100
   **b.** 10                **d.** 1,000          ____

**28.** The process through which oxygen is subtracted or hydrogen is added to a substance via a chemical reaction is:
   **a.** reduction         **c.** ionization
   **b.** oxidization       **d.** combustion          ____

**29.** Any substance that occupies space and has mass is:
- **a.** an atom
- **b.** an element
- **c.** matter
- **d.** a reaction

____

**30.** Characteristics that can only be determined by a chemical change in the substance are:
- **a.** chemical properties
- **b.** elemental properties
- **c.** molecular properties
- **d.** physical properties

____

**31.** A chemical combination of matter in definite proportions is a(n):
- **a.** atomic substance
- **b.** combined substance
- **c.** miscible substance
- **d.** pure substance

____

**32.** A physical combination of matter in any proportions is a:
- **a.** chemical mixture
- **b.** combined mixture
- **c.** physical mixture
- **d.** pure mixture

____

**33.** The _____ is the smallest chemical component of an element.
- **a.** anion
- **b.** atom
- **c.** cation
- **d.** molecule

____

**34.** Rapid oxidation of a substance, accompanied by the production of heat and light, is:
- **a.** reduction
- **b.** emulsification
- **c.** ionization
- **d.** combustion

____

**35.** Characteristics that can be determined without a chemical reaction and that do not involve a chemical change in the substance, are:
- **a.** chemical properties
- **b.** elemental properties
- **c.** molecular properties
- **d.** physical properties

____

# CHAPTER 13 Basics of Electricity

## MULTIPLE CHOICE

1. The flow of electricity along a conductor is called a(n):
   a. electric charge
   b. electric current
   c. energy swirl
   d. spark _____

2. Electric wires are usually covered with a rubber substance that is used as a(n):
   a. insulator
   b. conductor
   c. circuit
   d. fuse _____

3. A _____ is a device that changes direct current to alternating current.
   a. rectifier
   b. circuit breaker
   c. converter
   d. fuse box _____

4. The term _____ refers to a rapid and interrupted current that flows in one direction then in the opposite direction.
   a. rectifier current
   b. alternating current
   c. active current
   d. direct current _____

5. The unit that measures the pressure or force that pushes the flow of electrons through a conductor is a(n):
   a. amp
   b. watt
   c. ohm
   d. volt _____

6. Which unit measures the resistance of an electric current?
   a. ohm
   b. watt
   c. amp
   d. volt _____

7. The device that prevents excessive current from passing through a circuit is called a(n):
   a. fuse
   b. battery
   c. kilowatt
   d. ampere _____

8. A switch that automatically interrupts or shuts off an electric current at the first indication of an overload is a(n):
   a. voltage regulator
   b. ampere current
   c. circuit breaker
   d. battery charger _____

9. The negative electrode of an electrotherapy device is called a(n):
   a. anode
   b. electron
   c. carbode
   d. cathode _____

10. A process that forces an alkaline product into the tissues from the negative toward the positive pole is called:
    a. cataphoresis
    b. anaphoresis
    c. iontophoresis
    d. microcurrent _____

11. Grounding completes a(n) _____ and carries the current safely away.
    a. electric charge
    b. electric circuit
    c. complete electric circuit
    d. microcurrent _____

12. All the electrical appliances you use should:
    a. be battery operated
    b. be UL certified
    c. have a two-prong plug
    d. be used near water _____

13. When using _____, the active electrode is the electrode used on the area to be treated.
    a. alternating current
    b. direct current
    c. electric current
    d. galvanic current _____

14. Microcurrent can be used to _____ and restore elasticity.
    a. decrease metabolism
    b. increase muscle tone
    c. reduce lymph circulation
    d. prevent acidic reactions _____

15. Only licensed professionals can use:
    a. hairdryers
    b. steamers
    c. light therapy equipment
    d. vaporizers _____

16. A wavelength is the distance between successive peaks of _____ waves.
    a. electric
    b. electromagnetic
    c. galvanic
    d. infrared _____

**17.** Invisible light is the light at either end of the _____ that is invisible to the naked eye.
  **a.** electromagnetic spectrum
  **b.** spectrum of radiance
  **c.** spectrum of radiation
  **d.** visible spectrum of light
  ____

**18.** UVC light:
  **a.** is the light often used in tanning beds
  **b.** has the longest wave of the UV light spectrum
  **c.** is often called the burning light
  **d.** is blocked by the ozone layer
  ____

**19.** Catalysts are substances that speed up:
  **a.** chemical reactions
  **b.** acidic reactions
  **c.** alkaline reactions
  **d.** photoxic reactions
  ____

**20.** All lasers work by a process known as selective:
  **a.** emission
  **b.** electrolysis
  **c.** photothermolysis
  **d.** photosynthesis
  ____

**21.** Constant and direct current, having a positive and negative pole, that produces chemical changes when it passes through the tissues and fluids of the body is known as _____ current.
  **a.** galvanic
  **b.** alternating
  **c.** electric
  **d.** conductive
  ____

**22.** An extremely low level of electricity that mirrors the body's natural electrical impulses is:
  **a.** minicurrent
  **b.** microcurrent
  **c.** milliampere
  **d.** internal current
  ____

**23.** A medical device that uses multiple colors and wavelengths of focused light to treat such conditions as excessive hair and spider veins is a(n):
  **a.** laser
  **b.** infrared light device
  **c.** intense pulse light
  **d.** light-emitting diode
  ____

**24.** The thermal or heat-producing current with a high rate of oscillation or vibration commonly used for scalp and facial treatments is called:
  **a.** Tesla light-emitting current
  **b.** ultraviolet light
  **c.** intense pulse light
  **d.** Tesla high-frequency current
  ____

**25.** A device that works by releasing light onto the skin to stimulate specific responses at precise depths of the skin tissue is a(n):

a. laser  
b. infrared light device  
c. intense pulse light  
d. light-emitting diode     ____

# CHAPTER 14 Principles of Hair Design

## MULTIPLE CHOICE

1. Wave pattern changes can be created or changed temporarily with styling tools and permanently with:
   - **a.** thermal styling
   - **b.** chemicals
   - **c.** zigzag partings
   - **d.** flat irons
   ____

2. For a client with gold skin tones, a _____ haircolor would be flattering.
   - **a.** contrasting
   - **b.** toned
   - **c.** warm
   - **d.** cool
   ____

3. In designing for clients with large or broad shoulders, the stylist should create styles with:
   - **a.** more volume
   - **b.** less volume
   - **c.** more length
   - **d.** darker colors
   ____

4. Balance is described as creating equal or appropriate proportions to provide:
   - **a.** width
   - **b.** symmetry
   - **c.** structure
   - **d.** space
   ____

5. When opposite sides of a hairstyle have different lengths or different volume and appear to have equal visual weight, it is considered to have _____ balance.
   - **a.** horizontal
   - **b.** diagonal
   - **c.** symmetrical
   - **d.** asymmetrical
   ____

6. A recurrent pattern of movement in a design is referred to as:
   - **a.** rhythm
   - **b.** harmony
   - **c.** focus
   - **d.** balance
   ____

7. The area of a design where the eye is drawn to first before traveling to the rest of the design is called the:
   - **a.** balance
   - **b.** axis
   - **c.** emphasis
   - **d.** apex
   ____

8. To offset or round out the features of a square facial shape, the aim would be to:
   - **a.** create the illusion of width in the forehead
   - **b.** add volume to the sides
   - **c.** make the face seem shorter
   - **d.** create volume between the temples and jaw
   ____

9. The _____ profile has a receding forehead and chin.
   a. concave
   b. circular
   c. straight
   d. convex
   ____

10. The triangular section that begins at the apex or high point of the head and ends at the front corners is called the:
   a. crown area
   b. bang area
   c. line area
   d. convex area
   ____

11. Design texture can be created temporarily with the use of:
   a. heat and/or wet styling techniques
   b. cold and/or wet styling techniques
   c. heat and/or dry styling techniques
   d. cold and/or dry styling techniques

12. Which of these is *not* a physical characteristic taken into account when designing an artistic and suitable hairstyle?
   a. body posture
   b. features
   c. age
   d. head shape
   ____

13. Left natural, _____ hair may not support many styling options.
   a. medium, straight
   b. coarse, straight
   c. fine, straight
   d. fine, wavy
   ____

14. Which type of hair offers the most versatility in styling?
   a. wavy, medium hair
   b. coarse, straight hair
   c. fine, wavy hair
   d. fine, coarse hair
   ____

15. For ease of styling, _____ hair is generally best cut short.
   a. curly, medium coarse
   b. curly, coarse
   c. extremely curly,
   d. very curly, fine
   ____

16. The _____ profile has a receding forehead and chin.
   a. concave
   b. convex
   c. straight
   d. wavy
   ____

17. For a client with _____, you should direct the hair back and away from the face at the temples.
   a. close-set eyes
   b. a large forehead
   c. a crooked nose
   d. wide-set eyes
   ____

**18.** For a client with a _____, the hair should be directed forward in the chin area.
- **a.** round jaw
- **b.** receding chin
- **c.** small chin
- **d.** large chin

____

**19.** For a client with a _____ nose, bring hair forward at the forehead, with softness around the face.
- **a.** wide, flat
- **b.** long, narrow
- **c.** small
- **d.** prominent

____

**20.** If a male client has _____, a fairly close-trimmed beard and mustache would be very thinning to the overall appearance.
- **a.** dark hair
- **b.** light hair
- **c.** a wide face and a large jaw
- **d.** a wide face and full cheeks

____

**21.** To create length and height in hair design, use:
- **a.** vertical lines
- **b.** horizontal lines
- **c.** transitional lines
- **d.** single lines

____

**22.** To create width in hair design, use:
- **a.** contrasting lines
- **b.** horizontal lines
- **c.** diagonal lines
- **d.** directional lines

____

**23.** Lines that may move in a clockwise or counterclockwise direction are _____ lines.
- **a.** curved
- **b.** horizontal
- **c.** single
- **d.** parallel

____

**24.** The lines known as _____ lines can be straight or curved.
- **a.** single
- **b.** vertical
- **c.** directional
- **d.** parallel

____

**25.** Lines with a definite forward or backward movement are _____ lines.
- **a.** transitional
- **b.** contrasting
- **c.** directional
- **d.** diagonal

____

**26.** The square face shape:
- **a.** is narrow at the temples
- **b.** has hollow cheeks
- **c.** is rounded at the jaw
- **d.** is narrow at the middle third of the face

____

27. The face shape featuring a narrow forehead, extreme width through the cheekbones, and a narrow chin is the:
    a. inverted-triangle
    b. diamond
    c. heart-shaped
    d. pear-shaped          ____

28. The _____ face shape features a narrow forehead, wide jaw, and wide chin line.
    a. triangular
    b. oblong
    c. round
    d. square          ____

29. The face shape featuring a wide forehead and narrow chin line is the:
    a. triangular
    b. inverted-triangle
    c. oblong
    d. diamond          ____

30. The _____ face shape features a long, narrow face with hollow cheeks.
    a. square
    b. triangular
    c. oblong
    d. round          ____

# 15 Scalp Care, Shampooing, and Conditioning

## MULTIPLE CHOICE

1. What is the primary purpose of a shampoo service?
   - **a.** to recommend additional products services
   - **b.** to cleanse the hair and scalp
   - **c.** to recommend
   - **d.** to analyze the scalp
   ____

2. Which of the following is classified as a universal solvent?
   - **a.** salt
   - **b.** soap
   - **c.** lye
   - **d.** water
   ____

3. Small amounts of chlorine can be added to water to:
   - **a.** kill bacteria
   - **b.** add minerals
   - **c.** soften the water
   - **d.** harden the water
   ____

4. The ingredients on shampoo are listed in what order?
   - **a.** from largest to smallest percentage
   - **b.** from smallest to largest percentage
   - **c.** in order of weight
   - **d.** alphabetical order
   ____

5. A pH-balanced shampoo has a pH in the range of:
   - **a.** 3.0 to 3.0
   - **b.** 4.5 to 5.5
   - **c.** 6.0 to 7.0
   - **d.** 7.5 to 8.5
   ____

6. Which of the following substances absorb moisture or promote the retention of moisture?
   - **a.** proteins
   - **b.** silicones
   - **c.** humectants
   - **d.** preservatives
   ____

7. A _____ is designed to penetrate the cortex and reinforce the hair shaft from within, to temporarily reconstruct the hair.
   - **a.** detangler
   - **b.** balancing treatment
   - **c.** color enhancer
   - **d.** protein conditioner
   ____

8. Which of the following is used after a scalp treatment and before styling to remove oil accumulation?
   - **a.** medicated scalp lotion
   - **b.** scalp astringent lotion
   - **c.** scalp conditioner
   - **d.** leave-in conditioner
   ____

9. Brushing of the hair should never be done prior to:
   a. chemical services
   b. shampoo services
   c. styling services
   d. conditioning services ____

10. The most highly recommended hairbrushes are those made from:
    a. nylon bristles
    b. plastic bristles
    c. natural bristles
    d. metal bristles ____

11. As a safety feature for the client, during a shampoo you should monitor the water temperature by:
    a. waiting for the client to direct you to make it warmer or cooler
    b. keeping one finger over the edge of the spray nozzle in contact with the water
    c. using the nozzle to spray your palms periodically
    d. dipping your elbow into the water in the sink every few minutes ____

12. A scalp treatment used when there is a deficiency of natural oil on the hair or scalp should contain:
    a. mineral oil base products
    b. sulfonated oil base products
    c. strong soap preparations
    d. moisturizers and emollient ingredients ____

13. High-frequency current should never be used on hair treated with tonics that contain:
    a. water
    b. alcohol
    c. oil
    d. conditioning agents ____

14. Excessive oiliness is caused by:
    a. clogged pores
    b. a fungus called malassezia
    c. overactive sebaceous glands
    d. inactive sebaceous glands____

15. When working a shampoo into a lather, you should use:
    a. the cushions of your
    b. your nails
    c. your palms fingertips
    d. the sides of your fingers ____

16. The primary difference between a relaxation massage and a treatment massage is:
    a. the duration of the massage
    b. the type of drape used
    c. your finger movements
    d. the products you use ____

17. What should be the primary consideration when selecting a shampoo?
    a. the condition of the client's hair and scalp
    b. the amount of money the client is willing to pay
    c. the type of shampoo you have the most of in stock
    d. the type of service you are planning to perform after the shampoo ____

18. Color-enhancing shampoos are used to:
    a. dull the color of the hair
    b. add a great deal of color to the hair
    c. add brassiness to the hair
    d. eliminate unwanted color tones from the hair ____

19. All of the following are types of conditioners *except*:
    a. leave-in                 c. treatment or repair
    b. rinse-out                d. spray-on ____

20. Spray-on thermal protectors safeguard against the harmful effects of _____ the hair.
    a. cutting                  c. conditioning
    b. shampooing               d. blowdrying ____

21. For a client with _____ hair, it is recommended that you use a gentle cleansing shampoo and a light leave-in conditioner.
    a. fine, damaged            c. curly, damaged
    b. fine, straight           d. curly, dry ____

22. Appropriate products for coarse, damaged, dry hair include all of the following *except*:
    a. deep-moisturizing shampoo for damaged hair
    b. leave-in conditioner
    c. spray-on thermal protector treatments
    d. deep-conditioning treatments and hair masks. ____

23. Part One of the Three-Part procedure includes:
    a. helping your client through the scheduling and payment process
    b. performing the actual service the client has requested
    c. cleaning and disinfecting your tools
    d. advising the client and promoting products ____

24. What is the correct way to rinse your implements after cleaning them?
    a. run them under warm flowing water
    b. run them under cold flowing water
    c. dip them into a tub of warm water
    d. dip them directly into disinfectant                     ____

25. You should wait until _____ before discussing your retail product recommendations.
    a. a blowdryer is operating        c. the client consultation
    b. the service is complete         d. the client has paid   ____

26. Rainwater or chemically softened water that contains only a small amount of minerals is called:
    a. soft water                      c. deionized water
    b. hard water                      d. sparkling water       ____

27. Water that contains minerals that reduce the ability of soap or shampoo to lather properly is called:
    a. soft water                      c. deionized water
    b. hard water                      d. distilled water       ____

28. A _____ procedure is one that may produce undesirable side effects.
    a. constrained                     c. contraindicated
    b. contradicted                    d. countermanded         ____

29. Shampoo containing special ingredients that are very effective in reducing dandruff or relieving other scalp conditions is called _____ shampoo.
    a. balancing                       c. medicated
    b. clarifying                      d. nonstripping          ____

30. Shampoo designed to make the hair appear smooth and shiny and to improve the manageability of the hair is called _____ shampoo.
    a. clarifying                      c. balancing
    b. conditioning                    d. medicated             ____

31. Shampoo containing an active chelating agent that binds to metals and removes them from the hair is called _____ shampoo.
    a. clarifying                      c. conditioning
    b. chelating                       d. balancing             ____

**32.** Shampoo designed to wash away excess oiliness while preventing the hair from drying out is called _____ shampoo.

    **a.** balancing               **c.** conditioning

    **b.** clarifying               **d.** medicated     ____

**33.** Shampoo that cleanses the hair without the use of soap and water is _____ shampoo.

    **a.** humectant               **c.** dry

    **b.** soft                    **d.** astringent     ____

**34.** The _____ end of a surfuctant molecule is water-attracting.

    **a.** lipophilic               **c.** hydrophilic

    **b.** humectant               **d.** astringent     ____

**35.** The _____ end of a surfuctant molecule is oil-attracting.

    **a.** humectant               **c.** astringent

    **b.** hydrophilic             **d.** lipophilic     ____

# CHAPTER 16 Haircutting

## MULTIPLE CHOICE

1. The reference point that signals a change in head shape from flat to round or vice versa is the:
   - **a.** crown area
   - **b.** occipital corner
   - **c.** four corners
   - **d.** parietal ridge
   ____

2. The straight lines used to build weight or create a one-length or low-elevation haircut are:
   - **a.** parallel lines
   - **b.** horizontal lines
   - **c.** weight lines
   - **d.** diagonal lines
   ____

3. The straight lines used to remove weight or create graduated layers are:
   - **a.** cutting lines
   - **b.** diagonal lines
   - **c.** vertical lines
   - **d.** horizontal lines
   ____

4. For control during haircutting, the hair is divided into uniform working areas called:
   - **a.** foundations
   - **b.** uneven
   - **c.** parts
   - **d.** sections
   ____

5. The angle at which the fingers are held when performing a haircut is the:
   - **a.** end shape
   - **b.** blunt cut
   - **c.** cutting line
   - **d.** perimeter line
   ____

6. Which guideline is used when creating layers or a graduated cut?
   - **a.** traveling guideline
   - **b.** outer guideline
   - **c.** stationary guideline
   - **d.** shape guideline
   ____

7. The technique of combing hair away from its natural falling position, rather than straight out from the head toward a guideline, is called:
   - **a.** subsectioning
   - **b.** overdirection
   - **c.** traveling guidelines
   - **d.** undercutting
   ____

8. For a client with a long face, the stylist would recommend a style that adds:
   a. volume and height on top
   b. fullness on the sides
   c. weight to the chin and front
   d. fullness in length                                             ____

9. To compensate for shrinkage associated with curly hair, the stylist should allow for shrinkage of:
   a. 1/2 inch to 2 inches          c. 1/3 inch to 1 inch
   b. 1/4 inch to 1 inch            d. 1 inch to 3 inches            ____

10. The direction that hair grows from the scalp into a natural falling position is the:
    a. outermost perimeter          c. parallel section
    b. fringe area                  d. growth pattern               ____

11. Which type of comb is used for close tapers in the scissors-over-comb technique?
    a. wide-toothed comb            c. tail comb
    b. barber comb                  d. styling comb                 ____

12. The technique used to free up the dominant cutting hand to cut a subsection is called:
    a. moving the shears            c. transferring the comb
    b. removing the shears          d. working the shears           ____

13. The term used to describe the pressure applied to hair when combing or holding a subsection is:
    a. tension                      c. elevation
    b. sectioning                   d. angle                        ____

14. When cutting hair, a general rule of thumb is to stand or sit:
    a. directly behind the area you are cutting
    b. directly in front of the area you are cutting
    c. to the right of the area you are cutting
    d. to the left of the area you are cutting                      ____

15. The technique of cutting below the fingers or inside the knuckles using a horizontal cutting line creates:
    a. uniform or increasing layers
    b. a high level layered effect or a bi-level cut
    c. a shorter layer haircut or a shag effect
    d. a blunt haircut or heavier graduated haircut                 ____

16. The visual line in a haircut, where the ends of the hair hang together, is the:
    a. guideline
    b. weight line
    c. graduated line
    d. stationary line ____

17. Parting a haircut in the opposite way it was cut to check for precision of line and shape is called:
    a. cross-checking
    b. consistent tension
    c. mirror elevation
    d. blunt cutting ____

18. For a blunt haircut, when using the wide teeth of a comb when cutting, comb the section first with the fine teeth and then:
    a. change the position of the comb and comb with fine teeth
    b. switch comb to alternate hand and comb with fine teeth
    c. turn the comb around and comb with the wide teeth
    d. turn the comb on its side and comb with fine teeth ____

19. The term used to describe how hair is moved over the head is:
    a. head form
    b. distribution
    c. fringe
    d. weight line ____

20. A method of cutting or thinning hair where the fingers and shears glide along the edge of the hair to remove length is:
    a. angle cutting
    b. razor cutting
    c. blunt cutting
    d. slide cutting ____

21. The process of removing excess bulk or cutting for effect without shortening hair length is known as:
    a. blunt cutting
    b. angle cutting
    c. texturizing
    d. compensating ____

22. Thinning hair to graduated lengths using a sliding movement with shear blades partially open is called:
    a. slithering
    b. notching
    c. point cutting
    d. angle cutting ____

23. When performing the slicing technique on the surface of the haircut, it is best to work on:
    a. damp hair
    b. soapy hair
    c. wet hair
    d. dry hair ____

24. When using the clipper-over-comb technique, the length is determined by the:
    **a.** apex of the head
    **b.** angle of the comb
    **c.** size of the section
    **d.** type of clipper used
    ____

25. Haircuts _____ have often reflected a change in the thinking of the time.
    **a.** in the last 50 years
    **b.** in the last 100 years
    **c.** throughout modern times
    **d.** throughout history
    ____

26. The ability to duplicate an existing haircut or create a new haircut from a photo will build a stronger professional relationship between the stylist and:
    **a.** vendors
    **b.** manager
    **c.** clients
    **d.** fellow stylists
    ____

27. Elevation creates:
    **a.** graduation and layers
    **b.** cutting lines
    **c.** casts and crowns
    **d.** shrinkage
    ____

28. The outer line of a cut is known as the:
    **a.** parameter
    **b.** guideline
    **c.** cutting line
    **d.** perimeter
    ____

29. Shears should be sharpened:
    **a.** whenever the sharpening technician comes to the salon
    **b.** only as needed
    **c.** every three months
    **d.** every six months
    ____

30. You should use _____ tension when your goal is to create precise lines.
    **a.** minimal
    **b.** maximum
    **c.** moderate
    **d.** zero
    ____

31. Using a razor on _____ hair will weaken the cuticle and cause frizzing.
    **a.** straight
    **b.** fine
    **c.** blond
    **d.** curly
    ____

32. A client consultation should be performed _____ every haircut.
    **a.** before
    **b.** after
    **c.** during
    **d.** before and after
    ____

33. The client's hair should be _____ before the consultation.
    a. uncleansed and styled
    b. uncleansed and unstyled
    c. cleansed and styled
    d. cleansed and unstyled ____

34. A quick way to analyze a face shape is to determine if it is:
    a. long or short
    b. wide or narrow
    c. wide or long
    d. narrow or long ____

35. A fine hair strand is much _____ than a coarse hair strand.
    a. fatter
    b. skinnier
    c. darker in color
    d. more difficult to cut ____

36. Hair density is the number of individual strands on _____ of scalp.
    a. 1/4 square inch
    b. 1/3 square inch
    c. 1/2 square inch
    d. 1 square inch ____

37. Clippers:
    a. are mainly used when creating long haircuts
    b. must never be used without a guard
    c. are mainly used to remove bulk from the hair
    d. may be used with guards of various lengths ____

38. Cast shears are usually _____ than forged shears.
    a. less expensive to purchase
    b. more expensive to produce
    c. easier to bend back into shape
    d. more dense ____

39. The _____ on a pair of shears is designed to give you more control over the shear.
    a. bumper
    b. thumb hole
    c. finger tang
    d. pivot & adjustment area ____

40. Your shears should be cleaned and lubricated once a:
    a. day
    b. week
    c. month
    d. year ____

41. Before purchasing a pair of shears, ensure that the company has authorized someone in your area to _____ the company's shears.
    a. clean
    b. lubricate
    c. polish
    d. sharpen ____

42. Knowing how to hold your tools properly will help you avoid muscle strain in your:
    a. legs
    b. shoulders
    c. chest
    d. arms _____

43. When palming the shears, you hold the comb with your _____ fingers.
    a. thumb, index, and middle
    b. index, middle, and ring
    c. middle, ring, and pinky
    d. thumb, middle, and pinky _____

44. When cutting hair, it is important to always use _____ tension.
    a. minimum
    b. moderate
    c. maximum
    d. consistent _____

45. Heavier graduated haircuts work well on hair that _____ when dry.
    a. contracts
    b. expands
    c. becomes curlier
    d. becomes shinier _____

46. Which of these statements about razor cutting is true?
    a. A shear cut gives a softer appearance than a razor cut.
    b. When working with a razor, the ends are cut at an angle.
    c. Shears have much finer blades than razors.
    d. When working with a razor, the line is blunt. _____

47. Texturizing *cannot* be done with:
    a. cutting shears
    b. thinning sheers
    c. a razor
    d. clippers _____

48. When using clippers, you should always work _____ the natural growth patterns, especially in the nape.
    a. in the direction of
    b. against
    c. across
    d. alternately with and against _____

49. When trimming a male client's facial hair, it is recommended that you check _____ and ask if he would like to you remove any excess hair.
    a. his ears
    b. his eyebrows
    c. both his ears and eyebrows
    d. neither his ears nor eyebrows _____

**50.** The term _____ refers to the shape of the head.
- **a.** head form
- **b.** skull form
- **c.** hairline
- **d.** guideline

_____

**51.** Spots that mark where the surface of the head changes are:
- **a.** four corners
- **b.** angles
- **c.** reference points
- **d.** perimeters

_____

**52.** The widest area of the head is the:
- **a.** occipital bone
- **b.** parietal ridge
- **c.** nape
- **d.** apex

_____

**53.** The bone that protrudes at the base of the skull is the:
- **a.** parietal ridge
- **b.** orbital bone
- **c.** occipital bone
- **d.** nape

_____

**54.** The highest point at the top of the head is the:
- **a.** apex
- **b.** peak
- **c.** pate
- **d.** nape

_____

**55.** The area at the back part of the neck is the:
- **a.** bevel
- **b.** cast
- **c.** notch
- **d.** nape

_____

**56.** The triangular section that begins at the apex and ends at the four corners is the:
- **a.** back area
- **b.** bang area
- **c.** bevel area
- **d.** cast

_____

**57.** A _____ is a thin continuous mark used as a guide.
- **a.** line
- **b.** head form
- **c.** layer
- **d.** part

_____

**58.** Lines parallel to the floor are _____ lines.
- **a.** vertical
- **b.** horizontal
- **c.** diagonal
- **d.** straight

_____

**59.** The space between two lines or surfaces that intersect at a given point is a(n):
- **a.** angle
- **b.** apex
- **c.** bevel
- **d.** cast

_____

**60.** Lines perpendicular to the floor are _____ lines.
- **a.** horizontal
- **b.** straight
- **c.** diagonal
- **d.** vertical

_____

**61.** Lines that have a slanting or sloping direction are
_____ lines.
   a. straight                    c. vertical
   b. horizontal                  d. diagonal          ____

**62.** The line dividing the hair at the scalp is a:
   a. part                        c. cast
   b. bevel                       d. graduation        ____

**63.** When creating uniform layers, the hair is elevated to
_____ degrees from the scalp and cut at the same
length.
   a. 180                         c. 60
   b. 90                          d. 45                ____

**64.** When hair contracts or lifts through the action of moisture
loss, the process is called:
   a. reduction                   c. contraction
   b. shrinkage                   d. parting           ____

# CHAPTER 17 Hairstyling

## MULTIPLE CHOICE

1. The first step in the hairstyling process should always be a:
   - **a.** cool water shampoo
   - **b.** draping procedure
   - **c.** client consultation
   - **d.** conditioning treatment ____

2. Shaping and directing the hair into an S formation using a comb, lotion, and the fingers is called:
   - **a.** hairstyling
   - **b.** finger waving
   - **c.** ridge curls
   - **d.** roller setting ____

3. In creating horizontal finger waves, the waves are placed:
   - **a.** up and down the head
   - **b.** on the heavy side of the head
   - **c.** down and parallel
   - **d.** sideways and parallel around the head ____

4. The stationary foundation of a pin curl is the:
   - **a.** base
   - **b.** curl
   - **c.** section
   - **d.** stem ____

5. Pin curls that produce tight, firm, long-lasting curls and allow for minimum mobility are known as:
   - **a.** off-base pin curls
   - **b.** half-stem pin curls
   - **c.** on-base pin curls
   - **d.** no-stem pin curls ____

6. Pin curls formed in a shaping should begin at the:
   - **a.** open end
   - **b.** closed side
   - **c.** odd side
   - **d.** shaping side ____

7. Pin curl bases are referred to as rectangular, triangular, square, or:
   - **a.** S-shaped
   - **b.** arc-based
   - **c.** no-base
   - **d.** circular ____

8. Pin curls sliced from a shaping and formed without lifting the hair from the head are known as:
   - **a.** stem curls
   - **b.** design curls
   - **c.** carved curls
   - **d.** ridge curls ____

9. The panel of hair on which a roller is placed is the:
   - **a.** stem
   - **b.** section
   - **c.** base
   - **d.** subsection ____

10. Hair between the scalp and the first turn of a roller is the:
    a. curl
    b. base
    c. arc
    d. stem ____

11. The point where curls of opposite directions meet forming a recessed area is called the:
    a. indentation
    b. convex
    c. divot
    d. wave ____

12. To smooth hair that is backcombed, the teeth of the comb or brush should be held at a _____ pointing away from you.
    a. 15-degree angle
    b. 45-degree angle
    c. 90-degree angle
    d. 0-degree angle ____

13. Which type of styling product is also commonly known as mousse?
    a. texturizer
    b. holding spray
    c. styling gel
    d. foam ____

14. A benefit of using _____ is that it offers firmer, longer hold for fine hair with the least amount of heaviness.
    a. heavy gel with weight
    b. holding spray
    c. texturizer
    d. pomade ____

15. Which of these styling aids is applied to damp wavy or curling hair to create a straight look when the hair is blown dry?
    a. foam
    b. straightening gel
    c. spray gel
    d. mousse ____

16. To remove dirt, oils, and product residue from the barrel of a thermal iron, use a dampened towel with a soapy solution containing a few drops of:
    a. styling gel
    b. peroxide
    c. ammonia
    d. conditioner ____

17. Which of the following is a technique used to temporarily straighten extremely curly or unruly hair until the hair is shampooed?
    a. hair pressing
    b. blowdrying
    c. thermal curling
    d. deep cleansing ____

18. Applying a thermal pressing comb through the hair twice on each side to remove curl is a:
    a. hard press
    b. soft press
    c. thermal press
    d. medium press
    ____

19. A tight scalp can be made more flexible with hair brushing and the systematic use of:
    a. conditioning masks
    b. scalp massage
    c. conditioning shampoos
    d. roller sets
    ____

20. When executing an updo, always inspect the shape you are building from every angle to ensure that it is:
    a. smooth and flat
    b. balanced and well-proportioned
    c. elaborate and sturdy
    d. soft and shiny
    ____

21. After heating the iron to the desired temperature, you test it on:
    a. the client's hair
    b. your own hair
    c. a piece of tissue paper
    d. your finger
    ____

22. When using rollers, one and a half turns will create:
    a. a wave
    b. curls
    c. a C-shape curl
    d. cornrows
    ____

23. Hot rollers are to be used on:
    a. wet hair only
    b. damp hair only
    c. dry hair only
    d. wet or dry hair
    ____

24. Clients are most likely to request a pleat for:
    a. a relaxing summer style
    b. a warming winter style
    c. casual activities
    d. a special event
    ____

25. How long do Velcro rollers need to stay in the hair?
    a. 5 to 10 minutes
    b. 10 to 15 minutes
    c. 15 to 20 minutes
    d. 20 to 30 minutes
    ____

26. Wrapping can be done:
    a. only on wet hair
    b. only on dry hair
    c. only on damp hair
    d. on wet or dry hair
    ____

27. The technique of drying and styling damp hair in one operation is called:
    a. shaping
    b. blowdry styling
    c. unistyling
    d. hair wrapping ____

28. The _____ is a nozzle attachment with a directional feature that creates a concentrated stream of air.
    a. volumizer
    b. stem
    c. diffuser
    d. concentrator ____

29. Thermal waving is also known as:
    a. thio waving
    b. straight waving
    c. Marcel waving
    d. shell waving ____

30. Nonelectrical thermal irons are commonly favored by stylists who cater to clients with _____ hair.
    a. straight
    b. wavy
    c. curly
    d. excessively curly ____

31. What is the best way to practice manipulative techniques with thermal irons?
    a. rolling the cold iron in your hand first forward, then backward
    b. rolling the cold iron in your hand first backward, then forward
    c. rolling the warmed iron in your hand first forward, then backward
    d. rolling the warmed iron in your hand first backward, then forward ____

32. Thermal curling is effective for all BUT which of the following?
    a. straight hair
    b. pressed hair
    c. wigs made of nylon hair
    d. wigs made of human hair ____

33. End curls can be used to give a finished appearance to the ends of _____ hair.
    a. long
    b. medium
    c. short
    d. long, medium, or short ____

34. Full-base curls:
    a. cannot be created with a thermal iron
    b. provide a strong curl
    c. provide little volume
    d. sit at the end of their base ____

35. Who can diagnose scalp skin disease?
    a. a dermatologist
    b. a cosmetologist
    c. a dermatologist or a cosmetologist
    d. neither a dermatologist nor a cosmetologist        ____

36. Coarse, extremely curly hair:
    a. requires extra heat to press
    b. requires little heat to press
    c. requires little pressure to press
    d. has a small diameter        ____

37. When tempering a new pressing comb, you should NOT:
    a. heat the comb until it is extremely hot
    b. coat the comb in petroleum or pressing oil
    c. cool the comb in a freezer
    d. rinse the comb under hot running water to remove the oil    ____

38. Which of the following is usually recommended at the side
    front hairline for a smooth, upsweep effect?
    a. barrel curls            c. cascade curls
    b. rectangular base curls  d. square base pin curls        ____

39. Which type of curls are usually recommended along the
    front or facial hairline to prevent breaks or splits in the
    finished hairstyle?
    a. ridge curls             c. triangular base pin curls
    b. cascade curls           d. rectangular base curls        ____

40. Which type of curls are suitable for curly hairstyles without
    much volume and lift, can be used on any part of the head,
    and will comb out with lasting results?
    a. ridge curls             c. rectangular base curls
    b. barrel curls            d. square base pin curls        ____

41. Where are skip waves typically found?
    a. the side of the head    c. the top of the head
    b. the back of the head    d. the forehead        ____

42. Pin curls placed immediately behind or below a ridge to
    form a wave are called:
    a. triangular base curls   c. barrel curls
    b. cascade curls           d. ridge curls        ____

**43.** Which type of curls are also known as stand-up curls?

    **a.** rectangular base curls     **c.** ridge curls

    **b.** cascade curls     **d.** triangular base pin curls   ____

**44.** Which type of curls have large center openings and are fastened to the head in a standing position on a rectangular base?

    **a.** cascade curls     **c.** barrel curls

    **b.** ridge curls     **d.** square base pin curls   ____

**45.** Which roller position is recommended for full volume?

    **a.** on base     **c.** half base

    **b.** off base     **d.** dual base   ____

**46.** Which roller position is recommended for the least volume?

    **a.** on base     **c.** half base

    **b.** off base     **d.** dual base   ____

**47.** Which of these is used to build a soft cushion or to mesh two or more curl patterns together for a uniform and smooth comb out?

    **a.** sidecombing     **c.** backcombing

    **b.** sidebrushing     **d.** backbrushing   ____

**48.** Which of these involves combing small sections of hair from the ends toward the scalp, causing shorter hair to mat at the scalp, forming a cushion or base?

    **a.** sidecombing     **c.** backcombing

    **b.** sidebrushing     **d.** backbrushing   ____

**49.** A _____ is a half-round, rubber-based brush.

    **a.** vent brush     **c.** classic styling brush

    **b.** grooming brush     **d.** teasing brush   ____

**50.** A _____ is generally an oval brush with a mixture of boar and nylon bristles.

    **a.** vent brush     **c.** classic styling brush

    **b.** grooming brush     **d.** teasing brush   ____

**51.** A _____ is a thin, nylon styling brush that has a tail for sectioning, along with a narrow row of bristles.

    **a.** vent brush     **c.** classic styling brush

    **b.** grooming brush     **d.** teasing brush   ____

52. A _____ is a brush used to speed up the blowdrying process.
   a. vent brush
   c. classic styling brush
   b. grooming brush
   d. teasing brush          ____

53. Finger waving was very popular during the:
   a. 1920s and 1930s
   c. 1960s and 1970s
   b. 1940s and 1950s
   d. 1980s and 1990s          ____

54. Arc-base pin curls are also known as:
   a. S-curls
   c. half-moon curls
   b. V-curls
   d. full-moon curls          ____

55. Which part of a roller curl is also known as the circle?
   a. the base
   c. the stem
   b. the curl
   d. the paddle          ____

56. How many times do you turn the roller to create a C-shape curl?
   a. one
   c. two
   b. one and a half
   d. two and a half          ____

57. Velcro rollers can be used:
   a. only on wet hair
   c. only on damp hair
   b. only on dry hair
   d. on wet, dry, or damp hair ____

58. A hood dryer is recommended if you want:
   a. a set that does not last long
   c. a softer result
   b. the hair to dry quickly
   d. pin curls          ____

59. When you use a comb with teeth spaced closely together, it:
   a. removes definition from the curl
   c. creates a textured surface
   b. lifts the hair away from the head
   d. creates a smooth surface          ____

60. Which type of styling product is also known as wax?
   a. pomade
   c. finishing spray
   b. silicone
   d. volumizer          ____

# CHAPTER 18 Braiding and Braid Extensions

## MULTIPLE CHOICE

1. In natural-hairstyling services, texture refers to all BUT which of the following qualities?
   a. the diameter of the hair
   b. the feel of the hair
   c. the length of the hair
   d. the wave pattern _____

2. Which of the following is recommended for a client with a square face?
   a. a style with more width at the sides
   b. a style with height
   c. using bangs or sweep braids across the forehead
   d. framing the face with longer braids _____

3. The _____ face is a too-long oval and requires a style with more width at the sides.
   a. pear-shaped
   b. elongated
   c. oval
   d. heart-shaped _____

4. Which brush is recommended for scalp stimulation and removal of dirt and lint from locks?
   a. vent brush
   b. boar-bristle brush
   c. nylon-bristle brush
   d. square paddle brush _____

5. Which of the following is a characteristic of Kanekalon?
   a. It closely mimics human hair
   b. It is not very durable
   c. It is not heat-resistant
   d. It is prone to tangling _____

6. When curly hair is braided wet, it _____ as it dries.
   a. falls apart
   b. remains unchanged
   c. expands
   d. shrinks _____

7. A(n) _____ braid is created using a three-strand underhand braid technique where strands are woven under the center strand.
   a. French
   b. inverted
   c. visible
   d. invisible _____

8. Single braids can move:
   a. in any direction
   b. from side to side
   c. up and down
   d. diagonally _____

9. Extensions for single braids are integrated into natural hair using the:
   a. two-strand overhand technique
   b. three-strand underhand technique
   c. individual braid technique
   d. medium to large techniques          ____

10. Which of the following is NOT a basic method of locking?
    a. the comb technique          c. the palm roll
    b. braids or extensions         d. the block roll          ____

11. In some African tribes, different styles of braiding indicated:
    a. a person's social status
    b. the family to which a person belonged
    c. whether the person had children
    d. whether the person was married          ____

12. What is the most important feature of the wide-toothed comb?
    a. the length of the teeth
    b. the distance between the teeth
    c. the material from which the comb is made
    d. the sharpness of the teeth          ____

13. Most human hair used for hair extensions is imported from which part of the world?
    a. South America          c. Eastern Europe
    b. Asia                    d. South Africa          ____

14. Blowdrying does NOT:
    a. soften the hair
    b. dry wet hair quickly
    c. make hair more manageable for combing
    d. tighten and shrink the wave pattern          ____

15. The fishtail braid is best done on:
    a. long, layered hair          c. long, non-layered hair
    b. short, layered hair         d. short, non-layered hair          ____

16. How long does a tree braiding service take?
    a. 1 hour          c. 6 hours
    b. 4 hours         d. 90 minutes          ____

17. During which developmental phase of locks can a bulb be felt at the end of each lock?
    a. sprouting stage
    b. growing stage
    c. prelock stage
    d. maturation stage
    ____

18. During which developmental phase of locks does the hair begin to regain length?
    a. sprouting stage
    b. growing stage
    c. prelock stage
    d. maturation stage
    ____

19. During the first developmental phase of locks, the hair coil:
    a. is rough in texture
    b. has a matte texture
    c. is straight
    d. has an open end
    ____

20. Which of these is a braid created with two strands that are twisted around each other?
    a. fishtail braid
    b. invisible braid
    c. rope braid
    d. single braid
    ____

21. Which of these are separate networks of curly, textured hair that have been intertwined and meshed together?
    a. French braids
    b. locks
    c. cornrows
    d. canerows
    ____

22. A _____ is used to dry hair without disturbing the finished look and without dehydrating the hair.
    a. hood dryer
    b. pick nozzle
    c. concentrator
    d. diffuser
    ____

23. The practice of overlapping two strands to form a candy cane effect is known as:
    a. twisting
    b. weaving
    c. plaiting
    d. inverting
    ____

24. When performing a braiding service, it is recommended that you use _____ to create shapes and finished looks, and to trim bangs and excess extension material.
    a. two-inch scissors
    b. three-inch scissors
    c. five-inch scissors
    d. eight-inch scissors
    ____

25. The term _____ refers to narrow rows of invisible braids that lie close to the scalp and are created with a three-stand, on-the-scalp braiding technique.
    a. cornrows
    b. locks
    c. twists
    d. dreadlocks
    ____

26. Which of these is a tool that separates the hair as it combs, and is recommended for detangling wet curly hair?
    a. finishing comb          c. tail comb
    b. double-toothed comb     d. cutting comb          ____

27. Which of these is a tool used for cutting small sections, and should only be used after the hair is softened and elongated with a blowdryer?
    a. finishing comb          c. tail comb
    b. double-toothed comb     d. cutting comb          ____

28. A _____ is recommended for lifting and separating textured hair.
    a. wide-toothed comb       c. pick with rounded teeth
    b. square paddle brush     d. vent brush            ____

29. A(n) _____ is a free-hanging braid with or without an extension that can be executed using either an underhand or an overhand technique.
    a. inverted braid          c. plait
    b. single braid            d. fishtail braid        ____

30. Which type of brush is recommended for releasing tangles, knots, and snarls in short, textured hair and long, straight hair?
    a. square paddle brush     c. vent brush
    b. boar-bristle brush      d. natural hairbrush     ____

31. What is the benefit of mixing yak hair with human hair?
    a. It makes the hair easier to color.
    b. It eliminates the need to wash the hair.
    c. It helps to remove the manufactured shine.
    d. It makes the hair easier to style.             ____

32. Which of these terms does NOT refer to a three-strand braid produced with an overhand technique?
    a. French braid            c. inverted braid
    b. invisible braid         d. rope braid            ____

33. The _____ method involves applying extensions to cornrows by building the braid up strand by strand.
    a. feed-in                 c. draw-down
    b. over-weave              d. button-through        ____

**34.** A finishing comb is usually _____ in length.
- **a.** 3 to 4 inches
- **b.** 5 to 6 inches
- **c.** 6 to 8 inches
- **d.** 8 to 10 inches

____

**35.** The flat leather pad with very close, fine teeth used to sandwich human hair extensions is called a:
- **a.** book board
- **b.** drawing board
- **c.** flat iron
- **d.** leather clamp

____

# 19 Wigs and Hair Additions

## MULTIPLE CHOICE

1. The fastest way to determine whether a strand of hair is synthetic is to:
   a. burn it with a match
   b. contact the manufacturer
   c. cut it with scissors
   d. wet and blowdry it
   ____

2. Which of the following is a disadvantage of synthetic hair?
   a. Synthetic hair always looks unnatural.
   b. Synthetic hair is more expensive than human hair.
   c. Synthetic hair cannot be exposed to extreme heat.
   d. Synthetic hair is more prone to fading.
   ____

3. When performing a haircutting procedure on a wig, the goal generally is to make the wig:
   a. fit more snugly
   b. more fashionable
   c. more comfortable
   d. look realistic
   ____

4. When cutting a wig using a free-form method, move from longer to shorter lengths, working:
   a. away from the weight
   b. toward the weight
   c. away from the forehead
   d. toward the forehead
   ____

5. Which method of construction is typically least expensive?
   a. hand-tied
   b. semi-hand-tied
   c. machine-made
   d. They are equally expensive.
   ____

6. When shampooing a wig, it is recommended that you avoid shampoos that have a(n):
   a. sulfur base
   b. oil base
   c. carbon base
   d. nitrogen base
   ____

7. Synthetic hair colors used on wigs and hairpieces are standardized according to the _____ colors on the haircolor ring used by wig and hairpiece manufacturers.
   a. 50
   b. 70
   c. 90
   d. 110
   ____

8. The _____ is a sewing stitch in which the thread is wound around the needle twice.
   a. double-lock stitch
   b. secure lock stitch
   c. overcast stitch
   d. loop stitch
   ____

9. The _____ involves attaching hair wefts or single strands with an adhesive or glue.
   a. track method
   b. lockstitch method
   c. sewing method
   d. bonding method
   ____

10. The fusion method of extensions requires that the bonding material be activated with:
    a. a liquid chemical activator
    b. a powdered chemical activator
    c. water
    d. heat
    ____

11. Which of these is NOT an advantage of using a hair addition made of human hair?
    a. It has greater durability.
    b. It has a more realistic appearance.
    c. It never frizzes or loses its curl in humid weather.
    d. It has the same styling and maintenance requirements as human hair.
    ____

12. When using heat on human hair, you should set the styling tool on:
    a. low
    b. medium
    c. high
    d. ultra high
    ____

13. Traditionally, brushes made with _____ bristles have been regarded as best for use on human hair.
    a. metal
    b. straw
    c. natural boar
    d. nylon
    ____

14. A hair wrap is secured to the client's own hair with:
    a. combs
    b. hairpins
    c. a bandana
    d. fast-drying adhesive
    ____

15. When sewing on an extension using the braid-and-sew attachment method, it is recommended that you do NOT use a _____ needle.
    a. straight
    b. custom-designed
    c. curved
    d. sharp
    ____

16. When bonding, it is recommended that you work
_____ away from the hairline to keep the wefts
from showing.
a. one half inch          c. one and one half inches
b. one inch               d. two inches                    ____

17. To use a linking method of attachment, the natural hair
should be at least how long?
a. 3 inches               c. 6 inches
b. 4 inches               d. 8 inches                      ____

18. A(n) _____ is a small wig used to cover the top
and crown of the head.
a. toupee                 c. cap wig
b. integration hairpiece  d. weft                          ____

19. A _____ is a long strip of hair with a threaded
edge.
a. bond                   c. root
b. block                  d. weft                          ____

20. A(n) _____ is a hairpiece that has openings in the
base, through which the client's own hair is pulled to blend
with the hair of the hairpiece.
a. semi-hand-tied wig     c. hair extension
b. integration hairpiece  d. capless wig                   ____

21. The head-shaped form on which a wig is secured for fitting,
coloring, and sometimes styling is known as a:
a. weft                   c. block
b. brand                  d. cap                            ____

22. A(n) _____ is a hair addition secured to the base
of the client's natural hair in order to add length, volume,
texture, or color.
a. hair extension         c. cap wig
b. toupee                 d. integration hairpiece          ____

23. A _____ is made by inserting individual strands of
hair into mesh foundations and knotting them with a needle.
a. cap wig                c. hand-tied wig
b. capless wig            d. machine-made wig               ____

**24.** Hair that has been shed from the head and gathered from a hairbrush is known as:
**a.** bonded hair
**b.** carved hair
**c.** turned hair
**d.** fallen hair

_____

**25.** A _____ is an artificial covering for the head consisting of a network of interwoven hair.
**a.** wig
**b.** weft
**c.** cap
**d.** block

_____

**26.** A wig constructed with an elasticized, mesh-fiber base to which the hair is attached is called a:
**a.** capless wig
**b.** cap wig
**c.** Remi wig
**d.** fusion bond

_____

**27.** Hair in which the root end of every single strand is sewn into the base is called:
**a.** bonded hair
**b.** carved hair
**c.** turned hair
**d.** fallen hair

_____

**28.** Which of the following is NOT an advantage of wigs made with synthetic hair?
**a.** They are a great value.
**b.** They always look natural.
**c.** They are often cut according to the latest styles.
**d.** They are available in nearly limitless colors.

_____

**29.** Indian hair is usually:
**a.** extremely curly
**b.** straight
**c.** tightly coiled
**d.** wavy

_____

**30.** When styling a wig, it is recommended that you:
**a.** use the wind test to gauge how realistic it looks
**b.** plaster the hair down
**c.** use a brush rather than your hands for a natural look
**d.** try to make it look perfect

_____

## MULTIPLE CHOICE

1. The chemical texture service that loosens overly curly hair into loose curls or waves is:
   a. curl softening
   b. curl re-formation
   c. alternate waving
   d. swelling compound
   ____

2. The layer of the hair that provides strength and elasticity is the:
   a. medulla
   b. regular
   c. cortex
   d. arrector
   ____

3. The natural pH of hair is:
   a. 4.0
   b. 5.0
   c. 7.0
   d. 8.0
   ____

4. In permanent waving, the size of the curl is determined by the:
   a. position of the rod
   b. length of the hair
   c. wrapping of the rod
   d. size of the rod
   ____

5. The technique of wrapping at a 90-degree angle or straight out from the center is:
   a. half off-base placement
   b. on-base placement
   c. off-base placement
   d. full-base placement
   ____

6. The two basic types of wrapping hair around a perm rod are the spiral method and:
   a. loop method
   b. croquignole method
   c. placement method
   d. horizontal method
   ____

7. A reduction reaction involves either the addition of hydrogen or removal of:
   a. oxygen
   b. peroxide
   c. carbon
   d. nitrogen
   ____

8. Most alkaline permanent waves have a pH between:
   a. 9.0 and 9.6
   b. 10.0 and 10.8
   c. 8.0 and 9.0
   d. 7.6 and 8.4
   ____

9. The basic components of acid waves are permanent wave solution, activator, and:
   a. conditioner
   b. stabilizer
   c. neutralizer
   d. shampoo
   ____

10. An endothermic wave must be activated using a(n):
    a. ammonia lotion          c. sulfite source
    b. outside heat source     d. reducing agent          ____

11. Permanent wave solution should be rinsed from the hair for
    a minimum of:
    a. 2 minutes               c. 15 minutes
    b. 10 minutes              d. 5 minutes               ____

12. The process of rearranging extremely curly hair into a
    straighter or smoother form is:
    a. chemical hair relaxing  c. continuation
    b. chemical smoothing      d. neutralizing            ____

13. Thio chemical relaxers usually have a pH value above:
    a. 5                       c. 9
    b. 10                      d. 6                       ____

14. Hydroxide ions left in the hair after a relaxer can be
    neutralized using a(n):
    a. acid-balanced shampoo   c. thio neutralizer
    b. conditioning rinse      d. acid-free shampoo       ____

15. Which type of relaxer contains one component and is used
    without any additional mixing?
    a. thio relaxers           c. metal hydroxide
                                  relaxers
    b. lye-based relaxers      d. acid-based relaxers     ____

16. Lithium hydroxide relaxers and potassium hydroxide
    relaxers are often advertised and sold as:
    a. conditioner relaxers    c. no chemical relaxers
    b. no-lye relaxers         d. lye relaxers            ____

17. Which type of bonds are relatively weak physical side
    bonds that are the result of an attraction between negative
    and positive electrical charges?
    a. disulfide bonds         c. salt bonds
    b. polypeptide bonds       d. waving bonds            ____

18. Which type of rod is also commonly known as a circle rod?
    a. loop rods               c. concave rods
    b. soft bender rods        d. straight rods           ____

**19.** For on-base placement, the hair is wrapped at a _____ angle beyond perpendicular to its base section, and the rod is positioned on its base.
a. 180-degree
c. 90-degree
b. 15-degree
d. 45-degree ____

**20.** Which of these permanent waves processes at room temperature?
a. ammonia-free wave
c. low-pH wave
b. exothermic wave
d. true acid wave ____

**21.** Chemical texturizers _____ the pH of the hair.
a. lower
c. neutralize
b. raise
d. do not affect ____

**22.** When should you perform an elasticity test?
a. before perming the hair
c. after perming the hair
b. while perming the hair
d. never ____

**23.** Porous hair:
a. is difficult to penetrate
b. should never be permed
c. can be damaged by a highly alkaline permanent waving solution
d. can be damaged by a highly acidic permanent waving solution ____

**24.** GMTG, the primary reducing agent in all acid waves, has:
a. no pH
c. a high pH
b. a neutral pH
d. a low pH ____

**25.** True acid waves:
a. have a pH between 5.5 and 8.0
c. process very quickly
b. require heat to process
d. produce a very firm curl ____

**26.** Ammonia-free waves:
a. have a very strong odor
c. contain some ammonia
b. are very acidic
d. can be damaging ____

**27.** In permanent waving, most of the processing takes place within:
a. 5 to 10 minutes
c. 20 to 30 minutes
b. 10 to 20 minutes
d. 45 to 60 minutes ____

**28.** With permanent waving, it is recommended that you:
   **a.** perm hair that has previously been treated with hydroxide relaxers
   **b.** perm excessively damaged hair
   **c.** examine the scalp before the perm service
   **d.** perform a test for metallic salts only if the client requests it ____

**29.** With extremely curly hair, the twists are the _____ sections of the hair stands.
   **a.** thickest and strongest
   **b.** thinnest and weakest
   **c.** thickest and weakest
   **d.** thinnest and strongest ____

**30.** Relaxers are:
   **a.** extremely alkaline
   **b.** extremely acidic
   **c.** mildly alkaline
   **d.** mildly acidic ____

**31.** If the client's hair has been treated with a hydroxide relaxer, it:
   **a.** has disulfide bonds that are in the process of reforming
   **b.** has strong disulfide bonds
   **c.** is ideal for permanent waving
   **d.** will not hold a curl ____

**32.** A _____ is a perm wrap in which one end paper is placed under and another is placed over the strand of hair being wrapped.
   **a.** double flat wrap
   **b.** double-rod wrap
   **c.** croquignole perm wrap
   **d.** single flat wrap ____

**33.** Which type of rods are usually about 12-inches (30.5 centimeters) long with a uniform diameter along the entire length?
   **a.** straight rods
   **b.** loop rods
   **c.** soft bender rods
   **d.** circle rods ____

**34.** Thioglycolic acid:
   **a.** has no odor
   **b.** is a common reducing agent
   **c.** is dark in color
   **d.** has a pleasant scent ____

**35.** The _____ is the innermost layer of the hair.
   **a.** cortex
   **b.** base
   **c.** medulla
   **d.** cuticle ____

36. The partings and bases radiate throughout the panels to follow the curvature of the head in which type of wrap?
    a. bricklay permanent wrap
    c. spiral perm wrap
    b. double flat wrap
    d. curvature permanent wrap
    ____

37. The chemical bonds that join amino acids together are called:
    a. hydrogen bonds
    c. disulfide bonds
    b. peptide bonds
    d. thio bonds
    ____

38. A _____ is a type of perm wrap in which the hair is wrapped at an angle other than perpendicular to the length of the rod.
    a. spiral perm wrap
    c. basic permanent wrap
    b. straight set wrap
    d. bookend wrap
    ____

39. Which of these is a method of hair straightening that combines the use of a thio relaxer with flat ironing?
    a. weave technique
    c. thio neutralization
    b. Japanese thermal straightening
    d. no-base relaxing
    ____

40. Which type of relaxer requires the application of a protective base cream to the entire scalp prior to the application of the relaxer?
    a. hydroxide relaxer
    c. thio relaxer
    b. metal hydroxide relaxer
    d. base relaxer
    ____

41. The middle layer of the hair is the:
    a. medulla
    c. cortex
    b. cuticle
    d. base
    ____

42. Which of these terms refers to the angle at which the rod is positioned on the head?
    a. base placement
    c. base insertion
    b. base direction
    d. base reduction
    ____

43. A _____ is a type of wrap that uses one end paper folded in half over the hair ends like an envelope.
    a. basic permanent wrap
    c. bricklay permanent wrap
    b. curvature permanent wrap
    d. bookend wrap
    ____

44. A _____ is a wrapping pattern in which all the rods within a panel move in the same direction and are positioned on equal-sized bases.
   a. basic permanent wrap
   c. double-rod wrap
   b. croquignole perm wrap
   d. bookend wrap _____

45. Which of these are commonly known as lye relaxers?
   a. metal hydroxide relaxers
   c. sodium hydroxide relaxers
   b. carbonate hydroxide relaxers
   d. iron hydroxide relaxers _____

46. Which rods are equal in diameter along their entire length or curling area?
   a. straight rods
   c. concave rods
   b. loop rods
   d. convex rods _____

47. Which of these terms refers to the thickness or thinness of a liquid?
   a. duration
   c. intensity
   b. viscosity
   d. amperage _____

48. The _____ is the tough exterior layer of the hair.
   a. cuticle
   c. base
   b. medulla
   d. cortex _____

49. Which of these terms refers to the position of the rod in relation to its base section?
   a. base altitude
   c. base direction
   b. half off-base placement
   d. base placement _____

50. A _____ is a type of wrap in which the hair is wrapped on one rod from the scalp to midway down the hair shaft.
   a. spiral perm wrap
   c. piggyback wrap
   b. double flat wrap
   d. bricklay permanent wrap _____

51. Which of these stops the action of the waving solution and rebuilds the hair into its new curly form?
   a. lanthionization
   c. hydroxide neutralization
   b. thio neutralization
   d. peptide neutralization _____

52. Long chains of amino acids joined together by peptide bonds are known as:
   a. neutralization chains
   c. amino chains
   b. monopeptide chains
   d. polypeptide chains _____

53. The process by which hydroxide relaxers permanently straighten hair is called:
    a. lanthionization
    b. permanent waving
    c. normalization
    d. disulfide bonding ____

54. Hydrogen bonds can be broken by:
    a. only water
    b. only heat
    c. either water or heat
    d. neither water nor heat ____

55. The reducing agent used in permanent waving solutions is commonly referred to as:
    a. hydroxide
    b. thio
    c. sulfate
    d. disulfide ____

56. Manufacturers add an alkalizing agent to waving solutions because the acid in them:
    a. swells the hair
    b. penetrates into the cortex
    c. both swells the hair and penetrates into the cortex
    d. neither swells the hair nor penetrates into the cortex ____

57. A pH of 7.0 is _____ than the pH of hair.
    a. 10 times more alkaline
    b. 100 times more alkaline
    c. 10 times more acidic
    d. 100 times more acidic ____

58. Most of the acid waves found in today's salons have a pH between:
    a. 7.8 and 8.2
    b. 9.5 and 10.5
    c. 3.8 and 4.2
    d. 4.5 and 5.5 ____

59. Which of these is NOT one of the three main components of an exothermic wave?
    a. permanent waving solution
    b. neutralizer
    c. activator
    d. concentrator ____

60. A(n) _____ uses an endothermic process.
    a. alkaline wave
    b. thio-free wave
    c. low-pH wave
    d. acid-balanced wave ____

61. Which type of perm is recommended for very damaged hair?
    a. true acid wave
    b. exothermic wave
    c. ammonia-free wave
    d. alkaline wave ____

62. What is the most common neutralizer?
    a. ammonia
    b. hydrogen peroxide
    c. sodium chloride
    d. distilled water        ____

63. When rinsing the hair for a permanent wave, it is recommended that you:
    a. never rinse for longer than 20 seconds
    b. make sure the hair is still moderately moist before neutralizing
    c. always smell the hair after the recommended time has elapsed
    d. aggressively blot the hair        ____

64. Japanese thermal straightening:
    a. is a recommended service for extremely curly hair
    b. usually takes about 30 minutes
    c. is appropriate for all color-treated hair
    d. is sometimes called thermal reconditioning        ____

65. Mild-strength relaxers are formulated for:
    a. normal hair texture with a medium natural curl
    b. fine, color-treated, or damaged hair
    c. very coarse, extremely curly hair
    d. resistant hair        ____

# CHAPTER 21 Haircoloring

## MULTIPLE CHOICE

1. The layer of the hair that provides strength and elasticity is the:
   - **a.** cortex
   - **b.** cuticle
   - **c.** follicle
   - **d.** medulla _____

2. In individual hair strands, hair texture is determined by the:
   - **a.** density
   - **b.** porosity
   - **c.** diameter
   - **d.** length _____

3. If the cuticle is lifted, allowing the hair to take color quickly, the hair is said to have:
   - **a.** average porosity
   - **b.** no porosity
   - **c.** low porosity
   - **d.** high porosity _____

4. Haircolor levels are arranged on a scale from:
   - **a.** 1 to 5
   - **b.** 1 to 10
   - **c.** 1 to 100
   - **d.** 0 to 14 _____

5. Hair color tones can be described as:
   - **a.** warm, neutral, or hot
   - **b.** warm, neutral, or cool
   - **c.** cool, neutral, or even
   - **d.** cool, warm, or primary _____

6. Colors that are described as sandy or tan are considered:
   - **a.** natural tones
   - **b.** primary tones
   - **c.** artificial tones
   - **d.** cool tones _____

7. Which color will help minimize orange tones in the hair?
   - **a.** violet
   - **b.** gold
   - **c.** green
   - **d.** blue _____

8. Pure or fundamental colors that cannot be achieved from a mixture are:
   - **a.** level colors
   - **b.** secondary colors
   - **c.** primary colors
   - **d.** cool colors _____

9. The strongest and only cool primary color is:
   - **a.** green
   - **b.** yellow
   - **c.** red
   - **d.** blue _____

10. Red added to blue-based colors will cause them to appear:
    **a.** lighter          **c.** golden
    **b.** darker           **d.** yellow          ____

11. A _____ color is achieved by mixing a secondary color and its neighboring primary color.
    **a.** warm             **c.** complementary
    **b.** tertiary         **d.** base            ____

12. Equal proportions of primary colors will produce:
    **a.** gray             **c.** brown
    **b.** white            **d.** green           ____

13. A primary and secondary color positioned opposite each other on the color wheel are considered:
    **a.** base colors      **c.** opposing colors
    **b.** tertiary colors  **d.** complementary colors   ____

14. Temporary color pigment molecules do not penetrate because they are:
    **a.** weak             **c.** neutral
    **b.** soft             **d.** large           ____

15. Semipermanent hair color on average should last:
    **a.** 4 to 6 days      **c.** 8 to 10 weeks
    **b.** 4 to 6 weeks     **d.** 2 to 3 weeks    ____

16. Which type of haircolor penetrates the hair shaft and is formulated to deposit but not lift color?
    **a.** demipermanent hair color   **c.** semipermanent color
    **b.** permanent hair color       **d.** semitemporary color   ____

17. Which type of haircolor lightens and deposits color at the same time and in a single process because it is more alkaline than no-lift deposit-only colors and is usually mixed with a higher-volume developer?
    **a.** temporary haircolor        **c.** semipermanent haircolor
    **b.** permanent haircolor        **d.** demipermanent haircolor ____

18. To provide maximum lift in a one-process color service, most high-lift colors require:
    **a.** 20-volume peroxide         **c.** 30-volume peroxide
    **b.** 15-volume peroxide         **d.** 40-volume peroxide     ____

19. During the decolorization process, natural hair can go through as many as:
    a. 2 stages
    b. 1 stage
    c. 10 stages
    d. 5 stages ____

20. Overlapping color can cause breakage and create a sign of roots or:
    a. uniform color
    b. a line of demarcation
    c. a barrier line
    d. streaking ____

21. The three forms of hair lighteners are:
    a. oil, powder, and cream
    b. oil, cream, and lotion
    c. powder, foam, and oil
    d. cream, powder, and foam ____

22. In _____, selected strands are picked up from a narrow section of hair with a zigzag motion of the comb, and lightener is applied only to these strands.
    a. slicing
    b. baliage
    c. free-form technique
    d. weaving ____

23. For clients with 80 to 100 percent gray, which haircolor is generally most flattering?
    a. a blond shade
    b. a medium-brown shade
    c. a dark-brown shade
    d. a red shade ____

24. To cover unpigmented hair in a salt-and-pepper client, the color formulation should be:
    a. one level darker than the natural level
    b. two levels lighter than the natural level
    c. four levels lighter than the natural level
    d. two levels darker than the desired level ____

25. The process of pretreating gray or very resistant hair to allow for better penetration is known as:
    a. formulating
    b. unpigmenting
    c. presoftening
    d. prelightening ____

26. On a lightener retouch, new growth is lightened:
    a. first
    b. second
    c. last
    d. not at all ____

27. To produce a haircolor that looks natural, how many primary colors must be present?
    a. one
    b. two
    c. three
    d. four ____

**28.** The best way to obtain pale blond results is to use:
  - **a.** temporary haircolor
  - **b.** pure bleach
  - **c.** single process blonding
  - **d.** double-process blonding ____

**29.** When hair is violet, it is recommended that you use _____ to balance it.
  - **a.** orange
  - **b.** green
  - **c.** yellow
  - **d.** red ____

**30.** When hair is blue, it is recommended that you use _____ to balance it.
  - **a.** orange
  - **b.** violet
  - **c.** red
  - **d.** green ____

**31.** Selecting _____ base colors creates brighter colors
  - **a.** cool
  - **b.** warm
  - **c.** neutral
  - **d.** a mix of cool and warm ____

**32.** Demipermanent haircolor _____ color.
  - **a.** both deposits and lifts
  - **b.** neither deposits nor lifts
  - **c.** lifts but does not deposit
  - **d.** deposits but does not lift ____

**33.** During a haircolor consultation, you should:
  - **a.** look at the client through the mirror
  - **b.** look at the client directly
  - **c.** look only at the client's hair
  - **d.** avoid looking at the client ____

**34.** Which of these words is the best choice to use when discussing haircolor with clients?
  - **a.** good
  - **b.** bleached
  - **c.** soft
  - **d.** frosted ____

**35.** When performing a patch test, which color should you use?
  - **a.** the same color that will be used for the haircolor service
  - **b.** a shade slightly darker than the client's natural shade
  - **c.** a shade slightly lighter than the client's natural shade
  - **d.** the lightest shade available ____

**36.** Hair that has previously received a color service will have:

**a.** no porosity                 **c.** a typical level of porosity
**b.** a greater degree of porosity    **d.** much less porosity   \_\_\_\_

**37.** Under-lightened hair is likely to appear to have more
_____ than the intended color.

**a.** violet or blue          **c.** red or green
**b.** orange or blue        **d.** yellow or orange   \_\_\_\_

**38.** The term _____, or hue, refers to balance of color.

**a.** shade               **c.** intensity
**b.** tone                **d.** level   \_\_\_\_

**39.** Which of these is a coloring technique that requires two
separate procedures in which the hair is prelightened before
the depositing color is applied?

**a.** cap technique         **c.** baliage
**b.** reverse highlighting    **d.** double-process
                                  application   \_\_\_\_

**40.** The melanin that gives blond and red colors to hair is
called:

**a.** eumelanin             **c.** pheomelanin
**b.** mixed melanin       **d.** cyanomelanin   \_\_\_\_

**41.** The powdered persulfate salts added to the haircolor to
increase its lightening ability are called:

**a.** activators             **c.** highlighters
**b.** toners               **d.** fillers   \_\_\_\_

**42.** The term _____ refers to a combination of equal
parts of a prepared permanent color mixture and shampoo
used the last five minutes and worked through the hair to
refresh the ends.

**a.** line of demarcation    **c.** oxidation
**b.** level system          **d.** soap cap   \_\_\_\_

**43.** Which of these terms refers to varying degrees of warmth
exposed during a permanent color or lightening process?

**a.** overtone              **c.** hue
**b.** contributing pigment    **d.** level   \_\_\_\_

**44.** Which of these is a technique of coloring strands of hair darker than the natural color?
a. reverse highlighting
b. two-step coloring
c. bleaching
d. highlighting
____

**45.** What is the unit of measurement used to identify the lightness or darkness of a color?
a. hue
b. tone
c. intensity
d. level
____

**46.** What is the proper way to write the term that refers to the natural color of hair?
a. haircolor
b. hair color
c. hair-color
d. hair/color
____

**47.** A(n) _____ is a chemical compound that lightens hair by dispersing, dissolving, and decolorizing the natural hair pigment.
a. toner
b. soap cap
c. lightener
d. activator
____

**48.** Which of these measures the concentration and strength of hydrogen peroxide?
a. intensity
b. volume
c. level
d. tone
____

**49.** Colors obtained from the leaves or bark of plants are called:
a. earth tone haircolors
b. biocolors
c. ecocolors
d. natural haircolors
____

**50.** A _____ is a nonammonia color that adds shine and tone to the hair.
a. gradual haircolor
b. pheomelanin
c. glaze
d. filler
____

**51.** The term _____ means difficult for moisture or chemicals to penetrate.
a. baliage
b. demipermanent
c. resistant
d. level
____

**52.** Which of the following is used to recondition damaged, overly porous hair and equalize porosity so that the hair accepts the color evenly from strand to strand and from scalp to ends?
a. conditioner filler
b. aniline derivatives
c. glaze
d. activator
____

53. Which of these is an oxidizing agent that, when mixed with an oxidation haircolor, supplies the necessary oxygen gas to develop the color molecules and create a change in natural haircolor?
   a. hydrogen peroxide developer
   b. permanent haircolor
   c. toner
   d. gradual haircolor
   ____

54. A _____ is used to equalize porosity and deposit color in one application to provide a uniform contributing pigment on prelightened hair.
   a. conditioner filler
   b. toning glaze
   c. color filler
   d. developer
   ____

55. Which of these is a process that involves taking a narrow, 1/8-inch (0.3 centimeters) section of hair by making a straight part at the scalp, positioning the hair over foil, and applying lightening or color?
   a. decolorizing
   b. baliage
   c. highlighting
   d. slicing
   ____

56. The system for understanding color relationships is called:
   a. the color wheel
   b. the law of color
   c. chromatics
   d. the rule of tones
   ____

57. The term _____ refers to the first time the hair is colored.
   a. virgin application
   b. proto-application
   c. pre-service
   d. retouch
   ____

58. Which type of melanin lends black and brown colors to hair?
   a. mixed melanin
   b. cyanomelanin
   c. pheomelanin
   d. eumelanin
   ____

59. A(n) _____ is a powdered lightener that cannot be used directly on the scalp.
   a. presoftener
   b. reverse highligher
   c. off-the-scalp lightener
   d. toner
   ____

60. Haircolors containing metal salts that change hair color gradually by progressive buildup and exposure to air, creating a dull, metallic appearance, are called:
   a. sodium haircolors
   b. gradual haircolors
   c. tertiary haircolors
   d. aniline derivatives
   ____

61. A _____ is a test performed to determine how the hair will react to the color formula and how long the formula should be left on the hair.
   a. strand test
   b. patch test
   c. base test
   d. activation test ____

62. When identifying natural levels for a haircolor service, your most valuable tool is the:
   a. finishing comb
   b. LED lamp
   c. vent brush
   d. color wheel ____

63. The medium primary color is:
   a. red
   b. blue
   c. yellow
   d. violet ____

64. Which type of color adds subtle color results?
   a. demipermanent color
   b. semipermanent color
   c. permanent haircolor
   d. temporary haircolor ____

65. Which of these is a role of the alkalizing ingredient in permanent haircolor?
   a. to decrease the penetration of the dye within the hair
   b. to prevent the lightening action of peroxide
   c. to raise the cuticle of the hair
   d. to coat the hair without penetrating it ____

66. Henna is an example of:
   a. metallic haircolor
   b. natural haircolor
   c. temporary haircolor
   d. highlighting haircolor ____

67. What is the standard hydrogen peroxide volume?
   a. 10-volume
   b. 20-volume
   c. 30-volume
   d. 40-volume ____

68. A release statement is NOT:
   a. designed to protect the school or salon for responsibility for accidents
   b. used to help explain to clients the risk involved in a chemical service
   c. required for most forms of malpractice insurance
   d. a legally binding contract ____

**69.** Semipermanent colors:

a. lighten color      c. deposit color

b. contain oxidizers      d. remove color    ____

**70.** A _____ consistency provides the best control during the application of lightener as part of a double-process haircoloring service.

a. creamy      c. powdery

b. watery      d. very thick    ____

# CHAPTER 22 Hair Removal

## MULTIPLE CHOICE

1. During the client consultation, all clients should complete a
   questionnaire that discloses _____ medications.
   - **a.** topical
   - **b.** oral
   - **c.** both oral and topical
   - **d.** neither oral nor topical    ____

2. An absolute requirement for laser hair removal is that the
   hair being removed must be:
   - **a.** lighter than the surrounding skin
   - **b.** darker than the surrounding skin
   - **c.** in the anagen phase
   - **d.** in the catagen phase    ____

3. In the nape area, the most common form of hair removal is
   usually performed using:
   - **a.** tweezers
   - **b.** electric clippers
   - **c.** shears
   - **d.** a straight razor    ____

4. The natural arch of the eyebrow follows the:
   - **a.** orbital bone
   - **b.** frontal bone
   - **c.** mandible bone
   - **d.** frontal muscle    ____

5. The recommended time between waxings is generally:
   - **a.** 1 week
   - **b.** 2 to 4 weeks
   - **c.** 4 to 6 weeks
   - **d.** 6 to 8 weeks    ____

6. If redness or swelling occurs after a waxing treatment,
   soothe the skin with the application of _____ and
   cool compresses.
   - **a.** aloe gel
   - **b.** a moisturizing lotion
   - **c.** rubbing alcohol
   - **d.** an astringent    ____

7. Which of these methods of hair removal is especially
   popular in Eastern cultures?
   - **a.** photoepilation
   - **b.** waxing
   - **c.** sugaring
   - **d.** threading    ____

8. An advantage of sugar waxing is that it can be used to
   remove hair as short as _____ long.
   - **a.** 1/8 inch
   - **b.** 1/4 inch
   - **c.** 1/2 inch
   - **d.** 1/3 inch    ____

9.  When hot wax is ready to be applied to the skin it should:
    a.  be bubbling from the heat
    b.  have a thick consistency, like peanut butter
    c.  flow off the spatula as a liquid
    d.  drip smoothly off the spatula        ____

10. If hot wax lands on the client in an area you do not wish to treat, you should remove it with:
    a.  a cloth saturated with warm water
    b.  a cloth saturated with rubbing alcohol
    c.  a lotion designed to dissolve wax
    d.  astringent or toner        ____

11. An epilator removes the hair from:
    a.  the bottom of the follicle      c.  the top of the follicle
    b.  the middle of the follicle      d.  all parts of the follicle        ____

12. Which method of hair removal uses intense light to destroy the growth cells of the hair follicles?
    a.  tweezing                        c.  electrolysis
    b.  photoepilation                  d.  hirsutism        ____

13. Which method of hair removal requires the removal of all the hair from the front and back of the bikini area?
    a.  sugaring                        c.  Brazilian bikini waxing
    b.  waxing                          d.  threading        ____

14. Which method of hair removal temporarily removes superfluous hair by dissolving it at the skin surface level?
    a.  threading                       c.  electrolysis
    b.  laser hair removal              d.  depilatory        ____

15. Which method of hair removal uses an electric current to destroy the growth cells of the hair?
    a.  photoepilation                  c.  laser hair removal
    b.  electrolysis                    d.  sugaring        ____

16. Which of the following is NOT a common contraindication for hair removal?
    a.  chronic migraines               c.  sunburn
    b.  recent cosmetic surgery         d.  pustules        ____

17. Which of these is NOT an area where men frequently request hair removal?
    a.  the neck                        c.  the chest
    b.  the feet                        d.  the back        ____

18. When performing a patch test for a depilatory, how long should you leave it on the skin?
    a. 30 to 60 seconds
    c. 5 to 7 minutes
    b. 2 to 3 minutes
    d. 7 to 10 minutes ____

19. Which of these is the appropriate hair removal procedure for a client's underarms?
    a. cutting with scissors
    c. waxing
    b. a depilatory
    d. tweezing ____

20. Tweezing is NOT an appropriate method of hair removal for which part of the body?
    a. the tops of the feet
    c. the bikini line
    b. the shoulders
    d. the upper lip ____

21. If hair is more than _____ long, it should be trimmed before waxing.
    a. 1/4 inch
    c. 1 inch
    b. 1/2 inch
    d. 1-1/2 inches ____

22. Which of these methods of hair removal is NOT an advanced technique that requires additional training and experience?
    a. threading
    c. sugaring
    b. Brazilian waxing
    d. tweezing ____

23. The condition known as hirsuties causes:
    a. unusual hair growth
    c. coarse hair
    b. premature baldness
    d. brittle hair ____

24. Electrolysis involves the administration of an electric current with a:
    a. set of round paddles
    c. needle-shaped electrode
    b. short metal strip
    d. rod-like electrode ____

25. Photoepilation:
    a. has significant side effects
    b. requires the use of needles
    c. poses a significant risk of infection
    d. can clear 50 to 60 percent of hair in 12 weeks ____

# 23 Facials

## MULTIPLE CHOICE

1. When removing a cleanser from the eye area, it should be done with damp facial sponges or cotton pads:
   a. in an upward and outward movement
   b. in down and across movements
   c. with back-and-forth movements
   d. in circular movements ____

2. When performing a skin analysis with a magnifying lamp, the first thing the technician should look for is the presence or absence of:
   a. closed comedones
   b. visible pores
   c. evaporated cells
   d. oily skin areas ____

3. Skin that has small pores and may be flaky or dry with fine lines and wrinkles is characterized as:
   a. dehydrated
   b. oily
   c. normal
   d. sensitive ____

4. Oily skin or skin that produces too much sebum may appear shiny or greasy and have:
   a. even pore distribution
   b. small pores
   c. flakes
   d. large pores ____

5. When a follicle becomes clogged, resulting in an infection of the follicle, it is caused by a type of acne bacteria called:
   a. hydrating bacteria
   b. sebumatic bacteria
   c. anaerobic bacteria
   d. aerobic bacteria ____

6. Red pimples that do not have a pus head are referred to as:
   a. elastin pimples
   b. acne papules
   c. pustules
   d. moles ____

7. Which of these is a skin condition caused by sun exposure or hormone imbalances resulting in dark blotches of color in areas of the skin?
   a. hypertrichosis
   b. acne
   c. dehydration
   d. hyperpigmentation ____

8. Which of these is a chronic hereditary disorder indicated by constant or frequent facial blushing is:
   a. rosacea
   b. tinea
   c. acne
   d. albinism ____

9. Cosmetology professionals are only allowed to use products that remove surface dead cells from the:
   a. subcutaneous tissue
   b. stratum dermis
   c. stratum corneum
   d. dermal layer ____

10. Which of these is a gentle chemical exfoliation acid that helps dissolve the bonds and intercellular cement between cells?
   a. alpha hydroxy acid
   b. emulsion acid
   c. astringent acid
   d. cryogenic acid ____

11. A _____ is a highly concentrated skin product applied under a moisturizer or sunscreen.
   a. gommage
   b. tonic
   c. mask
   d. serum ____

12. The thin, open-meshed, woven cotton fabric used in a paraffin mask application is called:
   a. mask padding
   b. microsilk
   c. gauze
   d. a pledget ____

13. Which massage movement involves the use of light continuous stroking movement with the fingers in a slow rhythmic manner?
   a. tapotement
   b. pétrissage
   c. kneading
   d. effleurage ____

14. Which of these is a form of pétrissage in which the tissue is grasped, gently lifted, and spread out?
   a. fulling
   b. rolling
   c. friction
   d. chucking ____

15. What is the most stimulating form of massage?
   a. fulling
   b. stroking
   c. tapotement
   d. chucking ____

16. The point on the skin over the muscle where pressure and stimulation will cause contraction of the muscle is referred to as the:
   a. insertion point
   b. motor point
   c. origin point
   d. connection point ____

17. When using a brushing machine to perform an exfoliation, the skin should be treated with a(n):
    a. thin layer of cleanser or moisturizer
    b. fairly thick layer of cleanser or moisturizer
    c. strong toner
    d. astringent lotion        ____

18. The process of softening and emulsifying hardened sebum stuck in the follicles is called:
    a. massage therapy          c. desincrustation
    b. passive therapy          d. electrotherapy        ____

19. Water-soluble products are penetrated into the skin using galvanic current and a process called:
    a. iontophoresis            c. cathodization
    b. micropenetration         d. extraction            ____

20. The therapeutic use of essential oils to enhance a person's physical and emotional well-being is:
    a. oil therapy              c. electrotherapy
    b. scentification           d. aromatherapy          ____

21. If you use harsh scrubs on sensitive skin, it can:
    a. aggravate redness        c. cause severe
       blistering
    b. possibly affect the      d. cause an infectious
       client's pacemaker          disease               ____

22. Sun-damaged skin is often confused with:
    a. sensitive skin           c. aging skin
    b. inflamed skin            d. hypopigmented skin     ____

23. Salon AHA exfoliants should never be used unless the client has been using 10 percent AHA products at home for _____ prior to the higher concentration salon treatment, and using a daily facial sunscreen product.
    a. at least one week        c. no more than one week
    b. at least two weeks       d. no more than two weeks ____

24. Compared to day-use products, night treatments are usually:
    a. lighter                  c. less intensive
    b. equal in strength and weight   d. more intensive  ____

**25.** One of the biggest benefits of massage is that it:
   **a.** causes clients' skin to tense, opening the pores
   **b.** eliminates the need for treatment products
   **c.** increases product absorption
   **d.** decreases the conditioning effect of treatment products  ____

**26.** Clay-based masks:
   **a.** cannot be used with other ingredients
   **b.** have an exfoliating effect
   **c.** do not dry on the skin
   **d.** make pores appear larger ____

**27.** Alginate masks are often _____-based.
   **a.** seaweed
   **b.** aloe
   **c.** sand
   **d.** vegetable  ____

**28.** Ingredients that attract water are known as:
   **a.** humectants
   **b.** fresheners
   **c.** serums
   **d.** astringents  ____

**29.** A(n) _____ is a follicle impacted with solidified sebum and dead cell buildup that appears as small bumps just underneath the skin's surface.
   **a.** ostium
   **b.** gommage
   **c.** open comedone
   **d.** closed comedone  ____

**30.** Which type of mask contains special crystals of gypsum?
   **a.** paraffin wax mask
   **b.** modelage mask
   **c.** cream mask
   **d.** friction mask  ____

**31.** Which of these terms refers to a lack of lipids?
   **a.** exfoliant
   **b.** couperose
   **c.** alipidic
   **d.** emollient  ____

**32.** Lotions that help rebalance the pH and remove remnants of cleanser from the skin are called:
   **a.** serums
   **b.** toners
   **c.** moisturizers
   **d.** exfoliants  ____

**33.** A(n) _____ is an applicator for directing the electric current from the galvanic machine to the client's skin.
   **a.** electrode
   **b.** amperage
   **c.** wringer
   **d.** ampoule  ____

34. The opening of a follicle is called a(n):
    a. anode
    b. hackle
    c. ostium
    d. folliclend ____

35. Which of these is a type of chemical exfoliant that works by dissolving keratin proteins in the surface cells of the skin?
    a. microdermabrasion
    b. tapotement
    c. desincrustation
    d. enzyme peel ____

36. A(n) _____ is an individual dose of serum contained in a small vial.
    a. ampoule
    b. cathode
    c. ostium
    d. anode ____

37. A(n) _____ is a follicle impacted with solidified sebum and dead cell buildup.
    a. closed comedone
    b. open comedone
    c. humectant
    d. pétrissage ____

38. Methods used to physically remove dead cell buildup are called:
    a. steamers
    b. electrodes
    c. mechanical exfoliants
    d. chemical exfoliants ____

39. The manual or mechanical manipulation of the body by rubbing, gently pinching, kneading, tapping, and other movements is called:
    a. telangiectasias
    b. massage
    c. iontophoresis
    d. microcurrent ____

40. Which of these terms refers to a condition that requires avoiding certain treatment procedures or products to prevent undesirable side effects?
    a. effleurage
    b. counter-treatment
    c. compensation
    d. contraindication ____

41. A(n) _____ is a peeling cream that is rubbed off on the skin.
    a. alpha hydroxy acid
    b. cleansing milk
    c. gommage
    d. humectant ____

42. Which of these is a condition characterized by distended or dilated surface blood vessels?
    a. telangiectasis
    b. iontophoresis
    c. albinism
    d. hyperpigmentation ____

43. Electrical treatments should NOT be performed on clients:
    a. who take isotretinoin
    b. who take Differin®
    c. with asthma
    d. with metal bone pins        ____

44. The cosmetologist should NOT wear which type of jewelry
    while administering a facial treatment?
    a. earrings
    b. rings
    c. a necklace
    d. an anklet        ____

45. Proper exfoliation will:
    a. make the skin more oily
    b. decrease the skin's
       moisture content
    c. decrease elasticity
    d. reduce hyperpigmentation        ____

46. Moisturizers for oily skin are most often in _____
    form.
    a. lotion
    b. gel
    c. powder
    d. spray        ____

47. Modelage masks:
    a. are recommended for oily skin
    b. increase blood circulation
    c. should be applied to the lower neck
    d. are appropriate for clients with claustrophobia        ____

48. When performing pétrissage:
    a. your movements should be confined to the face and
       neck
    b. you should apply a great deal of pressure
    c. you lift, squeeze, and press the tissue
    d. your movements should be jerky        ____

49. Which type of massage involves grasping the flesh firmly
    in one hand and moving the hand up and down along the
    bone while the other hand keeps the arm or leg in a steady
    position?
    a. wringing
    b. chucking
    c. rolling
    d. tapotement        ____

50. Hacking is performed with which part of the hands?
    a. the fingertips
    b. the backs
    c. the palms
    d. the edges        ____

# CHAPTER 24 Facial Makeup

## MULTIPLE CHOICE

1. A _____ foundation provides heavier coverage and is usually intended for dry skin types.
   a. water-based
   b. cream
   c. powder
   d. gel ____

2. Makeup should be blended onto the skin with:
   a. a spatula
   b. a disposable makeup sponge
   c. cotton balls
   d. a reusable brush ____

3. A _____ color is lighter than the client's skin tone and may have any finish.
   a. base
   b. contour
   c. medium
   d. highlight ____

4. To clean professional makeup brushes, a gentle shampoo or brush solvent is used, and the brush is placed into running water with the ferrule:
   a. pointing outward
   b. pointing upward
   c. pointing downward
   d. removed ____

5. To create a tertiary color you mix equal amounts of a secondary color and:
   a. its neighboring primary color on the color wheel
   b. its opposite primary color on the color wheel
   c. another secondary color
   d. its complementary color ____

6. Which eye color is considered neutral and can wear any makeup color?
   a. green
   b. blue
   c. brown
   d. hazel ____

7. The best type of lighting for color evaluation in the salon consultation area is:
   a. incandescent light
   b. LED light
   c. fluorescent light
   d. natural light ____

8. A(n) _____ face has greater length in proportion to its width than the square or round face.
   a. triangle-shaped
   b. diamond-shaped
   c. oblong-shaped
   d. pear-shaped ____

9. To minimize a short, flat nose, a lighter foundation is applied:
   a. on the cheeks and sides of the nose, ending at the tip
   b. down the center of the nose, ending at the tip
   c. on the sides of the nose and nostrils
   d. onto the sides of the nose and into the laugh lines of the face    ____

10. In eyebrow arching, the highest part of an eyebrow arch should be from the outer circle of the iris:
    a. upward
    b. to the outer corner of the eye
    c. to the outer corner of the nose
    d. to the middle of the nose ____

11. When red is _____ -based, it is cool.
    a. orange
    b. yellow
    c. gold
    d. blue    ____

12. The use of _____ minimizes prominent features so they are less noticeable.
    a. highlights
    b. shadows
    c. bright colors
    d. bright shades    ____

13. What is the goal of effective makeup application?
    a. to cover up any wrinkles or blemishes
    b. to remake the client's image according to an ideal standard
    c. to add a great deal of color to the client's face
    d. to enhance the client's individuality    ____

14. If the client has close-set eyes, it is recommended that you lightly apply shadow:
    a. up from the top of the eyes
    b. inward toward the nose from the inner edge of the eyes
    c. up from the outer edge of the eyes
    d. down from the lower edge of the eyes    ____

15. If the client has a square face, it is recommended that you
    a. create a high arch on the ends of the eyebrows
    b. make the eyebrows almost straight
    c. widen the distance between the eyebrows
    d. trim the outer edges of the eyebrows    ____

16. Which type of cosmetic is used to outline and emphasize the eyes?
    a. mascara
    c. eyeliner
    b. blush
    d. eye shadow
    ____

17. Which of these is a thick, heavy type of foundation used to hide dark eye circles, dark splotches, and other imperfections?
    a. face powder
    c. cake makeup
    b. concealer
    d. greasepaint
    ____

18. Heavy makeup used for theatrical purposes is known as:
    a. cake makeup
    c. concealer
    b. foundation
    d. greasepaint
    ____

19. Which of these is also known as base makeup?
    a. foundation
    c. cheek color
    b. color primer
    d. lip liner
    ____

20. The most common use of _____ outside the theater is to cover scars and pigmentation defects.
    a. color primer
    c. mascara
    b. cake makeup
    d. face powder
    ____

21. Which of these is used primarily to add a natural-looking glow to the cheeks?
    a. greasepaint
    c. foundation
    b. color primer
    d. blush
    ____

22. Which of these is a cosmetic preparation used to darken, define, and thicken the eyelashes?
    a. eye shadow
    c. mascara
    b. eyeliner
    d. concealer
    ____

23. Which of these is applied to the skin before foundation to cancel out and help disguise skin discoloration?
    a. color primer
    c. cheek color
    b. cake makeup
    d. face powder
    ____

24. Which of these is a cosmetic applied on the eyelids to accentuate or contour them?
    a. mascara
    c. eyeliner
    b. eye shadow
    d. blush
    ____

**25.** A _____ is a mineral or color agent from which a pigment is derived.
- **a.** tone
- **b.** lake
- **c.** blot
- **d.** matte

____

**26.** Cosmetic products that cause the formation of clogged pores are called:
- **a.** acneic
- **b.** pustulic
- **c.** comedogenic
- **d.** noncomedogenic

____

**27.** Loose powder is applied with a large powder brush or a:
- **a.** linen facecloth
- **b.** wooden pusher
- **c.** cotton swab
- **d.** cotton ball

____

**28.** Oil-based eye makeup removers are generally _____ with a small amount of fragrance added.
- **a.** mineral oil
- **b.** olive oil
- **c.** canola oil
- **d.** a water solution

____

**29.** Which type of brush has fine, tapered, firm bristles and is used to apply liquid liner or shadow to the eyes.
- **a.** angle brush
- **b.** concealer brush
- **c.** eyeliner brush
- **d.** brow brush

____

**30.** Which type of lashes are separate artificial eyelashes that are applied to the eyelids one at a time?
- **a.** strip lashes
- **b.** individual lashes
- **c.** band lashes
- **d.** strand lashes

____

# 25 Manicuring

## MULTIPLE CHOICE

1. A manicuring table lamp should use a _____ incandescent bulb or a fluorescent bulb.
   a. 10- to 30-watt
   b. 40- to 60-watt
   c. 70- to 90-watt
   d. 100- to 120- watt ____

2. Fine-grit abrasives are designed for removing very fine scratches and:
   a. buffing and polishing
   b. smoothing and refining
   c. aggressive buffing
   d. shortening and shaping ____

3. It takes approximately _____ to properly clean and disinfect implements after each use.
   a. 10 minutes
   b. 20 minutes
   c. 30 minutes
   d. 60 minutes ____

4. Nail products should be removed from their containers using a:
   a. wooden pusher
   b. finger
   c. plastic or metal spatula
   d. cotton swab ____

5. Which of the following products is designed to loosen and dissolve dead tissue from the nail plate?
   a. moisturizing lotion
   b. non-acetone remover
   c. acetone remover
   d. cuticle remover ____

6. Success in nail polish application is achieved by using four coats including:
   a. two coats of polish color and two top coats
   b. two base coats, one coat of polish color, and one top coat
   c. one base coat, two coats of polish color, and one top coat
   d. one base coat, one coat of polish color, and two top coats ____

7. A standard manicuring table:
   a. is usually 16 to 21 inches wide
   b. is usually 24 to 36 inches long
   c. has no drawers or shelves
   d. does not require cleaning and disinfection ____

8. If a single client is going to have both a manicure and a pedicure, how many pairs of gloves will the cosmetologist need?
   a. none
   b. one
   c. two
   d. three ____

9. Disinfection containers must have:
   a. a drain
   b. a tray
   c. a drain
   d. a lid ____

10. Which of the following is NOT kept in a supply tray?
    a. polishes
    b. gloves
    c. creams
    d. polish removers ____

11. Reusing implements without properly cleaning and disinfecting them is against the law in:
    a. California, New York, and Oregon
    b. every state but Virginia
    c. every state but Ohio
    d. all states ____

12. The best terry cloth towels for use in a personal service are:
    a. white
    b. gray
    c. yellow
    d. black ____

13. Soap is known to remove _____ of pathogenic microbes from the hands, when hand washing is performed properly.
    a. nearly 50 percent
    b. about 75 percent
    c. over 80 percent
    d. over 90 percent ____

14. Compared to non-acetone removers, acetone removers:
    a. work more quickly but are poorer solvents
    b. work less quickly but are poorer solvents
    c. work more quickly and are better solvents
    d. work less quickly but are better solvents ____

15. Which of the following is designed to seal the surface of the skin?
    a. nail oil
    b. nail cream
    c. nail lotion
    d. acetone ____

16. Which of the following is NOT a term used to describe a colored coating applied to the natural nail plate?
    a. nail lacquer
    b. nail varnish
    c. nail bleach
    d. nail enamel ____

17. Nail hardeners can be applied:
    a. only before the base coat
    b. only as a top coat
    c. either before the base coat or as a top coat
    d. neither before the base coat nor as a top coat ____

18. Blended oils:
    a. should only be mixed by those who have studied aromatherapy
    b. are not intended to target any specific response from the client
    c. should not be used because they are unpleasant for the client
    d. are commonly added to products such as body lotion and masks ____

19. Paraffin wax is:
    a. typically heated in a microwave
    b. a petroleum by-product that holds moisture in the skin
    c. applied to the client's skin in block form
    d. pleasant for the client, but frequently ruins nail enhancements ____

20. A spa manicure requires extensive knowledge of:
    a. nail care
    b. skin care
    c. both nail and skin care
    d. neither nail nor skin care ____

21. Which of these terms refers to the tools used to perform your services?
    a. implements
    b. instruments
    c. equipment
    d. prods ____

22. Which of these terms refers to age spots caused by UV radiation?
    a. hypotension
    b. hypertension
    c. hypopigmentation
    d. hyperpigmentation ____

23. Which massage movement involves a succession of strokes in which the hands glide over an area of the body with varying degrees of pressure or contact?
    a. pétrissage
    b. effleurage
    c. tapotement
    d. vibration ____

24. Rubbing a file across the sharp edge of another file to prepare it for use is called:
    a. file prepping
    b. sharpening
    c. filing
    d. buffing _____

25. Which implement is used to carefully trim away dead skin around the nails?
    a. metal pusher
    b. tweezers
    c. nippers
    d. nail clippers _____

26. Which massage movement involves rapid tapping or striking motions of the hands against the skin?
    a. friction
    b. pétrissage
    c. effleurage
    d. tapotement _____

27. Which implement is used to shorten the free edge quickly and efficiently?
    a. nippers
    b. nail clippers
    c. nail file
    d. buffer _____

28. Which method of massage incorporates various strokes that manipulate or press one layer of tissue over another?
    a. vibration
    b. tapotement
    c. effleurage
    d. friction _____

29. A service cushion:
    a. must be fully covered by a fresh, clean towel
    b. must, by law, be provided for the client during a manicure service
    c. is higher on the ends and lower in the middle
    d. is placed behind the client's back during a manicure _____

30. The wooden pusher is NOT used to:
    a. remove cuticle tissue from the nail plate
    b. remove implements from disinfectant solutions
    c. clean under the free edge of the nail
    d. apply products _____

31. Nail conditioners are primarily used to:
    a. thin out the nail plate
    b. soften the skin around the nails
    c. reduce brittleness
    d. add shine to the nail _____

32. The _____ nail has a square free edge that is rounded off at the corner edges.
    a. pointed
    b. squoval
    c. square
    d. oval _____

**33.** The round nail:
   **a.** is best suited to thin hands with long fingers and narrow nail beds
   **b.** should be highly tapered
   **c.** is completely straight across the free edge
   **d.** should extend just a bit past the fingertip ____

**34.** The _____ nail is a conservative shape that is thought to be attractive on most women's hands.
   **a.** oval          **c.** squoval
   **b.** pointed       **d.** square ____

**35.** When applying an iridescent or frosted polish, you must use strokes that are:
   **a.** crisscrossed over one another **c.** parallel to the sidewalls
   **b.** perpendicular to the sidewalls **d.** wavy ____

# 26 Pedicuring

## MULTIPLE CHOICE

1. When performing a pedicure, you should grasp the foot between your thumb and fingers at the:
   - **a.** bottom of the foot
   - **b.** heel area
   - **c.** mid-tarsal area
   - **d.** ankle area
   ____

2. What are the basic steps to properly disinfect a foot spa after each pedicure service?
   - **a.** Drain and remove water and contaminants, add soap and water, rinse, and dry.
   - **b.** Drain and remove water and contaminants, clean surface, disinfect with approved disinfectant, rinse, and dry.
   - **c.** Drain and remove water, disinfect with approved disinfectant, rinse, and dry.
   - **d.** Change water, add soap, disinfect with approved disinfectant, thoroughly rinse, and dry.
   ____

3. The weekly maintenance procedure for a pipe-less foot spa requires the disinfectant solution to remain in the foot spa:
   - **a.** at least 10 minutes
   - **b.** no more than 30 minutes
   - **c.** overnight
   - **d.** over the weekend
   ____

4. Which massage technique is used most with a pedicure?
   - **a.** effleurage
   - **b.** pétrissage
   - **c.** tapotement
   - **d.** reflexology
   ____

5. Which of the following should never be placed in the foot bath with the client's feet?
   - **a.** solution
   - **b.** antiseptic
   - **c.** magnesium salt
   - **d.** disinfectant
   ____

6. The chair a cosmetologist uses when performing a pedicure:
   - **a.** is usually high off the ground
   - **b.** should not be ergonomic
   - **c.** must be inexpensive
   - **d.** must be comfortable
   ____

7. Electric foot mitts:
   - **a.** provide a great deal of client relaxation
   - **b.** create a cooling effect on the feet
   - **c.** prevent mask ingredients from penetrating too deeply
   - **d.** are designed to be used without any other products
   ____

8. Exfoliating scrubs:
   a. are designed to dry greasy feet
   b. help reduce calluses
   c. are usually oil-based
   d. are smooth lotions ____

9. In order to be on time, you must be polishing
   _____ after beginning a one-hour pedicure.
   a. 10 to 15 minutes
   b. 30 to 35 minutes
   c. 45 to 50 minutes
   d. 50 to 55 minutes ____

10. Reflexology practitioners believe that pressing certain reflex
    points on the feet:
    a. transmit positive energy
    b. decrease blood flow
    c. cause significant discomfort
    d. reverse the signs of aging ____

11. A paraffin bath:
    a. stimulates circulation
    b. reduces product absorption
    c. increases inflammation
    d. cools the skin ____

12. Repeated exposure to pedicure water can cause:
    a. hyperpigmentation
    b. overhydration of the skin
    c. cracking on the hands
    d. a latex allergy ____

13. If a client books a standard pedicure and you discover that
    the feet are in unusually bad condition and will require more
    time than was scheduled, it is recommended that you:
    a. take as much time as necessary, even if it means that
       other clients must wait
    b. send the client home and tell her to book a longer
       appointment next time
    c. cancel the next few appointments to make time for the
       client
    d. tell the client you will do your best but that an additional
       appointment will be necessary ____

14. Scaly feet commonly require _____ treatment in
    the salon.
    a. daily
    b. weekly
    c. monthly
    d. yearly ____

15. Massage given during manicures and pedicures focuses on:
    a. draining lymphatic fluid
    b. muscle stimulation
    c. pain relief
    d. relaxation ____

16. Which of these implements is commonly known as a paddle?
    a. foot file
    b. nail rasp
    c. curette
    d. nail file
    ____

17. Which of these is a metal implement with a grooved edge used for filing and smoothing the edges of the nail plate?
    a. nail clipper
    b. nippers
    c. nail rasp
    d. curette
    ____

18. A _____ is a small scoop-shaped implement used for more efficient removal of debris from the nail folds, eponychium, and hyponychium areas.
    a. nail rasp
    b. curette
    c. nail brush
    d. tweezer
    ____

19. The best type of _____ have jaws that are straight and come to a point.
    a. nippers
    b. toenail clippers
    c. nail rasps
    d. nail brushes
    ____

20. Which implement is used to trim tags of dead skin?
    a. nippers
    b. nail clippers
    c. finishing scissors
    d. curette
    ____

21. How long are masks typically left on the client's skin?
    a. 5 to 10 minutes
    b. 10 to 15 minutes
    c. 15 to 20 minutes
    d. 20 to 30 minutes
    ____

22. If a client drifts off during a pedicure, it is recommended that you:
    a. try to engage her in pleasant conversation
    b. start telling her about the home care products that you offer
    c. leave her alone and let her enjoy the service
    d. squeeze her foot gently to wake her up
    ____

23. Clients should be warned not to shave their legs _____ a pedicure.
    a. 24 hours after
    b. 48 hours after
    c. 24 hours before
    d. 48 hours before
    ____

**24.** Some improvements in the feet require more than one appointment in services referred to as a:
   **a.** set
   **c.** series
   **b.** system
   **d.** symposium    ____

**25.** Who bears the responsibility for ensuring that proper disinfection of the pedicure bath occurs?
   **a.** the technician
   **b.** the salon
   **c.** neither the salon nor the technician
   **d.** both the salon and the technician    ____

# 27 Nail Tips and Wraps

CHAPTER

## MULTIPLE CHOICE

1. A _____ is a plastic, pre-molded form adhered to the natural nail to add length or support a nail enhancement product.
   - **a.** nail wrap
   - **b.** nail tip
   - **c.** nail overlay
   - **d.** nail adhesive
   ____

2. The shallow depression area of a nail tip is the:
   - **a.** well
   - **b.** contact
   - **c.** applicator
   - **d.** gelled
   ____

3. When applying nail tips to the natural nail plate, it is recommended that you use the _____ technique.
   - **a.** stop, hold, and release
   - **b.** stop, rock, and hold
   - **c.** rock, hold, and free
   - **d.** rock, slide, and release
   ____

4. When blending a nail tip at the contact area, the fine-grit buff block should be held:
   - **a.** at a 45-degree angle against the nail plate
   - **b.** at a 80-degree angle against the nail plate
   - **c.** at a 15-degree angle against the nail plate
   - **d.** flat across the surface of the nail plate
   ____

5. The strongest material used as a nail wrap is:
   - **a.** silk
   - **b.** paper
   - **c.** fiberglass
   - **d.** linen
   ____

6. The product that accelerates the curing process of resins and adhesives is called a wrap resin accelerator or:
   - **a.** heat spike
   - **b.** extender
   - **c.** activator
   - **d.** dehydrator
   ____

7. A product applied to the surface of natural nails to remove moisture and improve adhesion is a:
   - **a.** nail blender
   - **b.** nail activator
   - **c.** nail adhesive
   - **d.** nail dehydrator
   ____

8. A fabric piece cut to completely cover a crack or break in a nail wrap is a:
   - **a.** stress strip
   - **b.** repair patch
   - **c.** rebalance batch
   - **d.** refill strip
   ____

9. To avoid damaging nail wraps when removing existing polish, use a(n):
   a. acetone remover
   b. oil accelerator
   c. resin softener
   d. non-acetone remover ____

10. An implement similar to a nail clipper, designed especially for use on nail tips, is a:
    a. tip nipper
    b. tip cutter
    c. stress cutter
    d. tip buffer ____

11. Fabric wraps are the most popular type of nail wrap because of their:
    a. durability
    b. color
    c. price
    d. glossy shine ____

12. Gel adhesives are sometimes referred to as:
    a. activator
    b. overlays
    c. resin
    d. dehydrators ____

13. Which wraps are made from a very thin synthetic mesh with a loose weave?
    a. fiberglass wraps
    b. silk wraps
    c. linen wraps
    d. paper wraps ____

14. Which wraps are made from a thin natural material with a tight weave that becomes transparent when wrap resin is applied?
    a. linen wraps
    b. fiberglass wraps
    c. paper wraps
    d. silk wraps ____

15. Which wraps are simple to use, but lack the strength of fabric wraps?
    a. linen wraps
    b. silk wraps
    c. paper wraps
    d. fiberglass wraps ____

16. Which type of wraps are made from a closely woven, heavy material?
    a. silk wraps
    b. linen wraps
    c. fiberglass wraps
    d. paper wraps ____

17. Nail tip adhesives are commonly available in all BUT which of the following forms?
    a. tube with a pointed applicator tip
    b. one-drop applicator
    c. brush-on
    d. spray-on ____

**18.** A client with nail wraps should come back to the salon about _____ after the original application for the first maintenance service.

   **a.** one week

   **b.** two weeks

   **c.** three weeks

   **d.** four weeks    ____

**19.** The structural correction of the nail during a nail wrap maintenance service to ensure its strength, shape, and durability is known as a(n):

   **a.** fill

   **b.** backfill

   **c.** rebalance

   **d.** activation    ____

**20.** To remove fabric wraps, you first soak them in acetone and then:

   **a.** slide them off with a wooden pusher

   **b.** scrub them off with steel wool

   **c.** cut them off with nippers

   **d.** cut them off with scissors    ____

# CHAPTER 28 Monomer Liquid and Polymer Powder Nail Enhancements

## MULTIPLE CHOICE

1. Acrylic (methacrylate) nail enhancements are created by combining monomer liquid with:
   - **a.** monomer powder
   - **b.** polymer powder
   - **c.** liquid powder
   - **d.** molecular powder   ____

2. As monomer liquid absorbs a polymer powder, the product formed at the tip of the brush is referred to as a:
   - **a.** cup
   - **b.** bead
   - **c.** dot
   - **d.** pledget   ____

3. The initiator added to polymer powder is:
   - **a.** benzoyl peroxide
   - **b.** catalyst peroxide
   - **c.** sodium hydroxide
   - **d.** hydrogen peroxide   ____

4. To prevent product contamination, a dappen dish should have:
   - **a.** a loosely fitted lid
   - **b.** a large opening
   - **c.** a tightly fitted lid
   - **d.** an evaporation lid   ____

5. The type of glove recommended for nail salon services is:
   - **a.** nylon polymer
   - **b.** hard plastic
   - **c.** latex polymer
   - **d.** nitrile polymer   ____

6. The bead of product for shaping the free edge should have a:
   - **a.** wet consistency
   - **b.** dry consistency
   - **c.** medium consistency
   - **d.** moist consistency   ____

7. Which types of primers are most often used today?
   - **a.** acid-based and acid-free primers
   - **b.** acid-based and nonacid primers
   - **c.** acid-based and dual acid primers
   - **d.** acid-free and nonacid primers   ____

8. When applying nail primer, the brush should hold enough product to treat how many nails?
   - **a.** one or two
   - **b.** two or three
   - **c.** three or four
   - **d.** four or five   ____

**9.** After a service, what should you do with used monomer liquid that has been removed from the original container?
   **a.** pour it back into the container   **c.** pour it into a paper towel
   **b.** pour it directly into a plastic bag   **d.** pour it down the drain   ____

**10.** The _____ is the area of the nail that has all of the strength.
   **a.** apex                      **c.** sidewall
   **b.** stress area               **d.** eponychium   ____

**11.** A properly-worn dust mask will protect you from:
   **a.** dust only                 **c.** both dust and vapors
   **b.** vapors only               **d.** neither dust nor vapors   ____

**12.** In the maintenance service:
   **a.** the nail is made thicker
   **b.** the entire nail enhancement is made thicker
   **c.** the apex of the nail is removed
   **d.** the entire nail enhancement is removed   ____

**13.** Which of these statements about catalysts is correct?
   **a.** Catalysts slow down chemical reactions between monomer liquid and polymer powder.
   **b.** Catalysts are added to monomer liquid to control the set time.
   **c.** Monomer liquid is added to a catalyst to control the set time.
   **d.** Catalysts work by preventing the initiators from activating.   ____

**14.** Polymer powder is available:
   **a.** only in clear form         **c.** in white and pink forms
   **b.** only in white              **d.** in many colors   ____

**15.** Which of these refers to one unit called a molecule?
   **a.** polymer                    **c.** initiator
   **b.** monomer                    **d.** catalyst   ____

**16.** Which of these is a substance formed by combining many small molecules into very long chain-like structures?
   **a.** apex                       **c.** monomer
   **b.** bead                       **d.** polymer   ____

**17.** A(n) _____ is a substance that starts the chain reaction that leads to the creation of very long polymer chains.

a. initiator
b. catalyst
c. reactor
d. concentrator

____

**18.** A _____ is a bead created using equal amounts of liquid and powder.

a. wet bead
b. dry bead
c. damp bead
d. medium bead

____

**19.** A _____ is a bead created using twice as much liquid as powder

a. damp bead
b. medium bead
c. dry bead
d. wet bead

____

**20.** A _____ is a bead created using one-and-a-half times more liquid than powder.

a. medium bead
b. damp bead
c. wet bead
d. dry bead

____

**21.** Which of these is placed under the free edge and is used to extend the nail enhancements beyond the fingertip for additional length?

a. sidewall
b. monomer brush
c. nail form
d. curing strut

____

**22.** The area where the natural nail grows beyond the finger and becomes the free edge is called the:

a. stress area
b. nail form
c. apex
d. lunula

____

**23.** The area on the side of the nail plate that grows free of its attachment to the nail fold is called the:

a. lunula
b. sidewall
c. free edge
d. apex

____

**24.** The term _____ refers to an entire family of thousands of different substances, all of which share important, closely related features.

a. nylon
b. polymer
c. polypeptide
d. acrylic

____

**25.** Polymerization is also known as:

a. applying
b. resolving
c. hardening
d. maintaining

____

**26.** Which of these abrasives would be MOST appropriate for final buffing?

a. 120 grit

b. 200 grit

c. 320 grit

d. 360 grit

_____

**27.** After a monomer liquid and polymer powder service, you should wipe the dappen dish with _____ before storing it in a dust-free location.

a. acetone

b. hydrogen peroxide

c. hot water

d. cold water

_____

**28.** Nail extension undersides should:

a. always jut straight out

b. always dip

c. match in length from nail to nail

d. have a rough texture

_____

**29.** The apex is usually:

a. oval shaped and located on the thumb-side of the nail

b. oval-shaped and located in the center of the nail

c. rectangular and located at the base of the nail

d. round and located beneath the nail

_____

**30.** Odorless products must generally be used with a _____ mix ratio.

a. dry

b. wet

c. damp

d. medium

_____

# CHAPTER 29 UV Gels

## MULTIPLE CHOICE

1. A(n) _____ is a short chain of monomers not long enough to be considered a polymer.
   - **a.** post-polymer
   - **b.** methacrylate
   - **c.** oligomer
   - **d.** resin ____

2. What is the most common UV lamp on the market?
   - **a.** 4-watt
   - **b.** 9-watt
   - **c.** 7-watt
   - **d.** 12-watt ____

3. UV gel products are usually packaged in opaque pots or:
   - **a.** glass jars
   - **b.** clear plastic bottles
   - **c.** plastic bags
   - **d.** squeeze tubes ____

4. The tacky surface left on the nail after a UV gel has cured is called the _____ layer.
   - **a.** inhibition
   - **b.** contour
   - **c.** adhesion
   - **d.** primary ____

5. A _____ is recommended to check and refine the nail contour for UV gel nails.
   - **a.** nonabrasive
   - **b.** fine abrasive
   - **c.** medium abrasive
   - **d.** harsh abrasive ____

6. Viscosity is the measurement of the _____ of a liquid.
   - **a.** weight
   - **b.** thickness
   - **c.** volume
   - **d.** opacity ____

7. Which of these products is designed specifically to improve adhesion of UV gels to the natural nail plate?
   - **a.** nail primer
   - **b.** nail adhesive
   - **c.** UV bonding gel
   - **d.** nail cleanser ____

8. Introducing air into the UV gel as you apply it to the fingernail will:
   - **a.** help prevent cracking
   - **b.** help the gel to cure more evenly
   - **c.** give the nail a shinier appearance
   - **d.** reduce the strength of the cured gel ____

9. Which of these is a thick-viscosity resin that allows the cosmetologist to build an arch and curve on a fingernail?
   a. UV building gel
   b. soft UV gel
   c. pigmented UV gel
   d. UV bonding gel ____

10. A _____ is a chemical in UV gel resins that initiates the polymerization reaction.
   a. chemoinitiator
   b. oligomer
   c. capacitor
   d. photoinitiator ____

11. Which of these is a type of gel used over the finished UV gel to create a high shine?
   a. UV gel polish
   b. UV gloss gel
   c. UV bonding gel
   d. UV building gel ____

12. Which of these is a type of UV gel that cannot be removed with a solvent?
   a. hard UV gel
   b. soft UV gel
   c. UV self-leveling gel
   d. UV gloss gel ____

13. Which type of UV gel is also known as soakable gel?
   a. UV building gel
   b. UV gel polish
   c. pigmented UV gel
   d. soft UV gel ____

14. UV gels:
   a. have a strong odor
   b. do not file easily
   c. can be easy to maintain
   d. are typically harder than monomer liquid and polymer powder nail enhancements ____

15. Pigmented UV gels may be:
   a. UV building gels
   b. UV self-leveling gels
   c. either UV building gels or UV self-leveling gels
   d. neither UV building gels nor UV self-leveling gels ____

16. Which of the following is NOT another term for UV gloss gel?
   a. sealing gel
   b. layer gel
   c. finishing gel
   d. shine gel ____

17. If a UV light unit has four lamps in it, and each lamp is 7-watts, it is known as a _____ light unit.
   a. 3-watt unit
   b. 7-watt unit
   c. 11-watt unit
   d. 28-watt unit ____

18. Different UV lamps produce greatly differing amounts of UV light. This is referred to as the UV lamp intensity or:
    a. concentration
    b. strength
    c. amperage
    d. occlusion

    _____

19. To help control the heat generated from the chemical reaction that occurs when UV gels cure, it is recommended that you:
    a. have clients insert their hands into the UV lamp very quickly
    b. have clients insert their hands into the UV lamp slowly
    c. spritz the nails with water before inserting them into the UV lamp
    d. blow on the nails while they cure

    _____

20. UV gel polish:
    a. thickens over time
    b. thins out over time
    c. does not dry
    d. does not shine

    _____

# CHAPTER 30 Seeking Employment

## MULTIPLE CHOICE

1. The typical independent salon has about _____ styling stations.
   a. 3
   b. 5
   c. 10
   d. 40          ____

2. Which type of salon shares a national name, consistent image, and business formula with salons in other locations?
   a. franchise salon
   b. day spa
   c. value-priced salon
   d. medical spa          ____

3. Making contact with salons and professionals to establish contacts in the beauty industry is called:
   a. interviewing
   b. marketing
   c. advertising
   d. networking          ____

4. After doing a salon site visit, it is important to send the salon representative a:
   a. copy of your employment portfolio
   b. cover letter
   c. thank-you note
   d. resume          ____

5. Which of these questions can a potential employer legally ask during an interview?
   a. How old are you?
   b. Are you authorized to work in the United States?
   c. What is your native language?
   d. What types of illnesses or disabilities do you have?          ____

6. When going over the directions for the exam, if there are things you do not understand, you should:
   a. try to figure it out on your own
   b. turn your test in and take the exam another day
   c. focus on the parts of the exam you do understand
   d. ask the examiner          ____

7. When answering a multiple choice question:
   a. if two choices are opposites, one is probably correct
   b. you should stop reading the choices when you see one that looks correct
   c. responses such as "all of the above" are usually not the correct choice
   d. you should never guess under any circumstances          ____

**8.** Which of these words is an example of an absolute?
  **a.** sometimes      **c.** equal
  **b.** never          **d.** good          ____

**9.** When taking the practical exam, it is recommended that you do all BUT which of the following?
  **a.** Observe other practical exams prior to taking yours if allowed to do so.
  **b.** Follow all infection control and safety procedures throughout the exam.
  **c.** Focus on what the other test candidates are doing as you work.
  **d.** Listen carefully to the instructions and follow them explicitly.          ____

**10.** To be successful in cosmetology, it is important to develop:
  **a.** technical skills
  **b.** communication skills
  **c.** both technical and communication skills
  **d.** neither technical nor communication skills          ____

**11.** When preparing your professional resume, it is recommended that you:
  **a.** make it about two pages long
  **b.** primarily focus on the schools you have attended
  **c.** omit information about your professional skills
  **d.** focus on information relevant to the position you are seeking          ____

**12.** The process of reaching logical conclusions by employing logical reasoning is called:
  **a.** intuition           **c.** postulating
  **b.** deductive reasoning  **d.** deciphering          ____

**13.** A(n) _____ is a written summary of a person's education and work experience.
  **a.** employment portfolio  **c.** cover letter
  **b.** employment agreement  **d.** resume          ____

**14.** The basic question or problem on an exam is known as a:
  **a.** stem      **c.** query
  **b.** response  **d.** post          ____

**15.** Which of these terms refers to understanding the strategies for successfully taking tests?

   **a.** work ethic           **c.** street-smart

   **b.** test-wise            **d.** deductive reasoning   ____

**16.** A(n) _____ is a collection of photos and documents that reflect your skills, accomplishments, and abilities in your chosen career field.

   **a.** resume            **c.** employment agreement

   **b.** cover letter         **d.** employment portfolio   ____

**17.** Who should ask questions during the interview?

   **a.** only the interviewer

   **b.** only the interviewee

   **c.** both the interviewer and the interviewee

   **d.** neither the interviewer nor the interviewee   ____

**18.** Which of the following is NOT an example of a good study habit?

   **a.** staying up late studying the night before a test

   **b.** reading content carefully

   **c.** developing a detailed vocabulary list

   **d.** organizing and reviewing handouts   ____

**19.** Having _____ means being committed to a strong code of moral and artistic values.

   **a.** motivation          **c.** enthusiasm

   **b.** integrity            **d.** a strong work ethic   ____

**20.** Which type of salon is MOST likely to offer extras such as five-minute head, neck, and shoulder massages as part of the shampoo?

   **a.** high-end image salon      **c.** booth rental salon

   **b.** mid-priced full-service salon  **d.** basic value-priced salon  ____

# CHAPTER 31 On the Job

## MULTIPLE CHOICE

1. It is recommended that you select which of these people as a role model?
   - **a.** a manager
   - **b.** another stylist in the salon
   - **c.** a client
   - **d.** a vendor
   ____

2. The number one thing to remember in a service business is that your work revolves around:
   - **a.** serving your clients
   - **b.** making a profit
   - **c.** making yourself happy
   - **d.** helping your coworkers
   ____

3. Which of these is NOT a standard method of compensation in the salon industry?
   - **a.** salary
   - **b.** commission
   - **c.** salary plus commission
   - **d.** salary minus tips
   ____

4. Being a good team player includes:
   - **a.** focusing on your own work
   - **b.** withholding your knowledge
   - **c.** refusing to be subordinate
   - **d.** striving to help
   ____

5. The common range for commissions is:
   - **a.** 15–25 percent
   - **b.** 20–30 percent
   - **c.** 25–60 percent
   - **d.** 50–80 percent
   ____

6. When is the best time to think about getting your client back into the salon?
   - **a.** before she gets to the salon
   - **b.** while she is still in the salon
   - **c.** just after she leaves the salon
   - **d.** several days after she leaves the salon
   ____

7. Which payment structure is often used to motivate employees to perform more services, thereby increasing their productivity?
   - **a.** salary plus commission
   - **b.** salary plus tips
   - **c.** hourly rate
   - **d.** weekly rate
   ____

8. The usual amount to tip is _____ of the total service ticket.
   - **a.** 10 percent
   - **b.** 15 percent
   - **c.** 20 percent
   - **d.** 25 percent ____

9. The practice of recommending and selling additional services to your clients is known as:
   - **a.** incentivizing
   - **b.** retailing
   - **c.** hard selling
   - **d.** ticket upgrading ____

10. The term _____ refers to the percentage of the revenue that the salon takes in from services performed by a particular cosmetologist.
    - **a.** salary
    - **b.** wage
    - **c.** commission
    - **d.** tip ____

11. Which of these terms refers to customers who are loyal to a particular cosmetologist?
    - **a.** client base
    - **b.** walk-ins
    - **c.** loyalists
    - **d.** personnel ____

12. A(n) _____ is a document that outlines all the duties and responsibilities of a particular position in a salon or spa.
    - **a.** employment agreement
    - **b.** resume
    - **c.** job description
    - **d.** rental agreement ____

13. The act of recommending and selling products to your clients for at-home use is known as:
    - **a.** soft selling
    - **b.** ticketing
    - **c.** wholesaling
    - **d.** retailing ____

14. Which of these strategies will help you to effectively meet your clients' needs?
    - **a.** Always put yourself first.
    - **b.** Be punctual.
    - **c.** Say whatever is necessary to make a sale.
    - **d.** Once you have a job, stop learning and focus solely on working. ____

15. A good job description outlines all BUT which of the following?
    - **a.** all of the employee's duties
    - **b.** all of the employee's responsibilities
    - **c.** the attitudes the employee is expected to have
    - **d.** the specifics of the individual employee's salary ____

16. Which of these is usually the best form of compensation for a new salon professional to start out?
    a. salary
    c. commission
    b. salary plus commission
    d. tips
    ____

17. If you default, it means that you:
    a. open a line of credit
    c. fail to pay back a loan
    b. are asked to leave your job
    d. pay your bills on time
    ____

18. Which of these is a recommended method of increasing your income?
    a. lowering your prices for services
    b. spending more money
    c. retailing less
    d. working more hours
    ____

19. To be a proficient salesperson, it is recommended that you do all BUT which of the following?
    a. Familiarize yourself with the features of the products you sell.
    b. Always use a hard sell approach.
    c. Ask the client questions that determine a need.
    d. Deliver your sales talk in a relaxed, friendly manner.
    ____

20. Which of the following is NOT a recommended method for expanding your client base?
    a. Rush through services so that you can see more clients each day.
    b. Send clients birthday cards with special offers inside.
    c. Start a business card referral program.
    d. Be reliable, positive, and respectful of clients.
    ____

# 32 The Salon Business

## MULTIPLE CHOICE

1. When preparing your business plan, it is often helpful to consult with an _____ to prepare your financial documents.
   a. interior designer
   b. attorney
   c. architect
   d. accountant _____

2. Another name for an individual owner with complete control of a business is:
   a. business partner
   b. stockholder
   c. sole proprietor
   d. manager _____

3. Supplies used in the daily business operation are considered:
   a. retail supplies
   b. consumption supplies
   c. consumer supplies
   d. inventory supplies _____

4. Supplies purchased by a salon with the intention of selling these products to clients are:
   a. retail supplies
   b. consumption supplies
   c. inventory supplies
   d. client supplies _____

5. When planning and constructing the best physical layout for a salon, the primary concern should be:
   a. color scheme
   b. salon furniture
   c. salon carpeting
   d. maximum efficiency _____

6. It should always be your top priority to meet which of these financial obligations?
   a. utility bills
   b. vendor bills
   c. payroll
   d. rent or mortgage _____

7. Which of these is considered the very best form of advertising for a salon?
   a. radio spots
   b. satisfied clients
   c. television ads
   d. newspaper ads _____

8. A(n) _____ is a benchmark that, once achieved, helps you realize your mission and your vision.
   a. assignment
   b. result
   c. obligation
   d. goal _____

9. When choosing a location for your business, you should select one that:
   a. offers easy access
   b. has limited parking
   c. is secluded
   d. has low traffic ____

10. What is the minimum number of stockholders allowed for a corporation to exist?
    a. 0
    b. 1
    c. 2
    d. 3 ____

11. If you operate your salon in a building that you own, it is recommended that you purchase all BUT which of these types of insurance?
    a. liability insurance
    b. malpractice insurance
    c. renter's insurance
    d. burglary insurance ____

12. Which of these terms refers to your staff or employees?
    a. personnel
    b. constituents
    c. clients
    d. creditors ____

13. Human resources covers all BUT which of the following concerns?
    a. what you can and cannot say when hiring someone
    b. what you must do when firing someone
    c. what you should do when you need to increase sales
    d. how you manage your employees ____

14. Booking appointments is primarily whose job?
    a. the cosmetologist
    b. the client
    c. the manager
    d. the receptionist ____

15. The first goal of every business should be to:
    a. maintain current clients
    b. attract new clients
    c. compensate employees fairly
    d. upgrade existing equipment ____

16. Which part of a business plan outlines management levels and describes how the business will be run?
    a. Financial Documents
    b. Organizational Plan
    c. Vision Statement
    d. Mission Statement ____

17. Which part of a business plan summarizes your plan and states your objectives?
    a. Salon Policies
    b. Marketing Plan
    c. Mission Statement
    d. Executive Summary _____

18. Which part of a business plan includes projected financial statements, actual statements, and financial statement analyses?
    a. Organizational Plan
    b. Vision Statement
    c. Financial Documents
    d. Salon Policies _____

19. Which part of a business plan ensures that all clients and employees are treated fairly and consistently?
    a. Salon Policies
    b. Financial Documents
    c. Executive Summary
    d. Organizational Plan _____

20. Which part of a business plan is a long-term picture of what the business is to become and what it will look like when it gets there?
    a. Vision Statement
    b. Mission Statement
    c. Salon Policies
    d. Marketing Plan _____

21. Which part of a business plan outlines all of the research obtained regarding the clients your business will target and their needs, wants, and habits?
    a. Organizational Plan
    b. Financial Documents
    c. Marketing Plan
    d. Executive Summary _____

22. Which part of a business plan includes the owner's résumé, personal financial information, legal contracts, and any other agreements?
    a. Executive Summary
    b. Salon Policies
    c. Financial Documents
    d. Supporting Documents _____

23. Which part of a business plan is a description of the key strategic influences of the business?
    a. Vision Statement
    b. Mission Statement
    c. Supporting Documents
    d. Marketing Plan _____

24. An agreement to buy an established salon should include all BUT which of the following?
    a. an agreement on future maintenance costs
    b. disclosure of the conditions of the facility
    c. a formal or informal employee agreement
    d. confirmation of the identity of the owner _____

**25.** Costs to create even a small salon in an existing space can range from _____ per square foot.

a. $5 to $15

b. $20 to $35

c. $30 to $80

d. $75 to $125

_____

## CHAPTER 1—HISTORY AND CAREER OPPORTUNITIES

| | | |
|---|---|---|
| 1. b | 6. d | 11. c |
| 2. a | 7. a | 12. b |
| 3. d | 8. d | 13. a |
| 4. c | 9. b | 14. c |
| 5. b | 10. b | 15. b |

## CHAPTER 2—LIFE SKILLS

| | | |
|---|---|---|
| 1. b | 6. b | 11. d |
| 2. c | 7. a | 12. b |
| 3. a | 8. d | 13. c |
| 4. d | 9. c | 14. b |
| 5. a | 10. a | 15. d |

## CHAPTER 3—YOUR PROFESSIONAL IMAGE

| | |
|---|---|
| 1. c | 6. b |
| 2. b | 7. c |
| 3. a | 8. a |
| 4. d | 9. c |
| 5. b | 10. b |

## CHAPTER 4—COMMUNICATING FOR SUCCESS

| | | | |
|---|---|---|---|
| 1. c | 6. a | 11. c | 16. b |
| 2. b | 7. c | 12. b | 17. a |
| 3. a | 8. b | 13. a | 18. c |
| 4. b | 9. a | 14. b | 19. a |
| 5. d | 10. d | 15. c | 20. d |

## CHAPTER 5—INFECTION CONTROL: PRINCIPLES AND PRACTICES

| | | | | |
|---|---|---|---|---|
| 1. a | 11. a | 21. c | 31. a | 41. a |
| 2. d | 12. d | 22. a | 32. a | 42. b |
| 3. a | 13. b | 23. b | 33. c | 43. c |
| 4. c | 14. a | 24. d | 34. a | 44. d |
| 5. b | 15. d | 25. a | 35. d | 45. c |
| 6. c | 16. b | 26. b | 36. b | 46. a |
| 7. a | 17. b | 27. d | 37. b | 47. b |
| 8. c | 18. a | 28. b | 38. d | 48. a |
| 9. b | 19. d | 29. c | 39. c | 49. d |
| 10. c | 20. b | 30. b | 40. b | 50. d |

## CHAPTER 5—INFECTION CONTROL: PRINCIPLES AND PRACTICES (*continued*)

| | | | | |
|---|---|---|---|---|
| 51. c | 56. d | 61. c | 66. c | 71. b |
| 52. b | 57. c | 62. b | 67. b | 72. c |
| 53. a | 58. a | 63. d | 68. d | |
| 54. b | 59. d | 64. d | 69. a | |
| 55. b | 60. b | 65. c | 70. c | |

## CHAPTER 6—GENERAL ANATOMY AND PHYSIOLOGY

| | | | | |
|---|---|---|---|---|
| 1. b | 14. b | 27. d | 40. c | 53. b |
| 2. c | 15. d | 28. d | 41. b | 54. d |
| 3. b | 16. a | 29. b | 42. d | 55. b |
| 4. c | 17. c | 30. c | 43. b | 56. d |
| 5. a | 18. b | 31. b | 44. c | 57. a |
| 6. a | 19. a | 32. c | 45. c | 58. c |
| 7. b | 20. d | 33. b | 46. b | 59. a |
| 8. d | 21. d | 34. a | 47. c | 60. d |
| 9. b | 22. b | 35. b | 48. c | 61. b |
| 10. c | 23. c | 36. c | 49. b | 62. c |
| 11. a | 24. b | 37. b | 50. d | 63. d |
| 12. b | 25. a | 38. d | 51. a | 64. b |
| 13. a | 26. b | 39. b | 52. b | 65. a |

## CHAPTER 7—SKIN STRUCTURE, GROWTH, AND NUTRITION

| | | | | |
|---|---|---|---|---|
| 1. b | 8. a | 15. b | 22. c | 29. b |
| 2. a | 9. c | 16. c | 23. b | 30. c |
| 3. c | 10. b | 17. d | 24. a | 31. b |
| 4. d | 11. a | 18. c | 25. a | 32. a |
| 5. a | 12. d | 19. b | 26. c | 33. b |
| 6. c | 13. c | 20. a | 27. d | 34. a |
| 7. a | 14. d | 21. d | 28. a | 35. d |

## CHAPTER 8—SKIN DISORDERS AND DISEASES

| | | | | |
|---|---|---|---|---|
| 1. d | 7. a | 13. c | 19. c | 25. b |
| 2. c | 8. b | 14. a | 20. b | 26. a |
| 3. a | 9. d | 15. b | 21. d | 27. a |
| 4. d | 10. b | 16. d | 22. b | 28. b |
| 5. a | 11. c | 17. c | 23. a | 29. c |
| 6. c | 12. d | 18. c | 24. d | 30. b |

## CHAPTER 9—NAIL STRUCTURE AND GROWTH

| | | | | |
|---|---|---|---|---|
| 1. c | 6. d | 11. c | 16. c | 21. a |
| 2. a | 7. c | 12. a | 17. a | 22. b |
| 3. b | 8. b | 13. c | 18. b | 23. d |
| 4. a | 9. a | 14. b | 19. c | 24. d |
| 5. b | 10. d | 15. d | 20. c | 25. c |

## CHAPTER 10—NAIL DISORDERS AND DISEASES

| | | | |
|---|---|---|---|
| 1. a | 6. d | 11. d | 16. a |
| 2. b | 7. c | 12. b | 17. c |
| 3. b | 8. c | 13. d | 18. a |
| 4. d | 9. b | 14. d | 19. d |
| 5. c | 10. c | 15. b | 20. c |

## CHAPTER 11—PROPERTIES OF THE HAIR AND SCALP

| | | | | |
|---|---|---|---|---|
| 1. b | 15. b | 29. b | 43. b | 57. d |
| 2. c | 16. a | 30. d | 44. d | 58. c |
| 3. a | 17. d | 31. c | 45. d | 59. b |
| 4. c | 18. c | 32. a | 46. a | 60. d |
| 5. b | 19. b | 33. d | 47. c | 61. a |
| 6. d | 20. d | 34. d | 48. a | 62. c |
| 7. c | 21. c | 35. c | 49. d | 63. d |
| 8. b | 22. d | 36. a | 50. c | 64. a |
| 9. c | 23. a | 37. a | 51. b | 65. d |
| 10. d | 24. c | 38. b | 52. c | 66. b |
| 11. b | 25. b | 39. d | 53. b | 67. a |
| 12. a | 26. a | 40. a | 54. a | 68. b |
| 13. a | 27. c | 41. d | 55. b | 69. a |
| 14. c | 28. d | 42. c | 56. c | 70. a |

## CHAPTER 12—BASICS OF CHEMISTRY

| | | | | |
|---|---|---|---|---|
| 1. c | 8. b | 15. a | 22. a | 29. c |
| 2. d | 9. b | 16. d | 23. b | 30. a |
| 3. b | 10. c | 17. a | 24. a | 31. d |
| 4. a | 11. d | 18. c | 25. d | 32. c |
| 5. c | 12. a | 19. c | 26. b | 33. b |
| 6. d | 13. d | 20. b | 27. b | 34. d |
| 7. a | 14. c | 21. d | 28. a | 35. d |

## CHAPTER 13—BASICS OF ELECTRICITY

| | | | | |
|---|---|---|---|---|
| 1. b | 6. a | 11. b | 16. b | 21. a |
| 2. a | 7. a | 12. b | 17. d | 22. b |
| 3. c | 8. c | 13. d | 18. d | 23. c |
| 4. b | 9. d | 14. b | 19. a | 24. d |
| 5. d | 10. b | 15. c | 20. c | 25. d |

## CHAPTER 14—PRINCIPLES OF HAIR DESIGN

| | | | | |
|---|---|---|---|---|
| 1. b | 7. c | 13. c | 19. d | 25. c |
| 2. c | 8. d | 14. a | 20. d | 26. d |
| 3. a | 9. d | 15. d | 21. a | 27. b |
| 4. b | 10. b | 16. b | 22. b | 28. a |
| 5. d | 11. a | 17. a | 23. a | 29. b |
| 6. a | 12. c | 18. b | 24. d | 30. c |

## CHAPTER 15—SCALP CARE, SHAMPOOING, AND CONDITIONING

| | | | | |
|---|---|---|---|---|
| 1. b | 8. b | 15. a | 22. c | 29. c |
| 2. d | 9. a | 16. d | 23. c | 30. b |
| 3. a | 10. c | 17. a | 24. a | 31. a |
| 4. a | 11. b | 18. d | 25. b | 32. a |
| 5. b | 12. d | 19. d | 26. a | 33. c |
| 6. c | 13. b | 20. d | 27. b | 34. c |
| 7. d | 14. c | 21. a | 28. c | 35. d |

## CHAPTER 16—HAIRCUTTING

| | | | | |
|---|---|---|---|---|
| 1. c | 14. b | 27. a | 40. b | 53. c |
| 2. b | 15. d | 28. d | 41. d | 54. a |
| 3. c | 16. b | 29. b | 42. d | 55. d |
| 4. d | 17. a | 30. b | 43. a | 56. b |
| 5. c | 18. c | 31. d | 44. d | 57. a |
| 6. a | 19. b | 32. a | 45. b | 58. b |
| 7. b | 20. d | 33. d | 46. b | 59. a |
| 8. b | 21. c | 34. c | 47. d | 60. d |
| 9. a | 22. a | 35. b | 48. b | 61. d |
| 10. d | 23. d | 36. d | 49. c | 62. a |
| 11. b | 24. b | 37. d | 50. a | 63. b |
| 12. c | 25. d | 38. a | 51. c | 64. b |
| 13. a | 26. c | 39. c | 52. b | |

## CHAPTER 17—HAIRSTYLING

| | | | | |
|---|---|---|---|---|
| 1. c | 13. d | 25. a | 37. c | 49. c |
| 2. b | 14. c | 26. d | 38. b | 50. b |
| 3. d | 15. b | 27. b | 39. c | 51. d |
| 4. a | 16. c | 28. d | 40. d | 52. a |
| 5. d | 17. a | 29. c | 41. a | 53. a |
| 6. a | 18. a | 30. d | 42. d | 54. c |
| 7. b | 19. b | 31. a | 43. b | 55. b |
| 8. c | 20. b | 32. c | 44. c | 56. a |
| 9. c | 21. c | 33. d | 45. a | 57. b |
| 10. d | 22. a | 34. b | 46. b | 58. d |
| 11. a | 23. c | 35. a | 47. d | 59. c |
| 12. b | 24. d | 36. a | 48. c | 60. a |

## CHAPTER 18—BRAIDING AND BRAID EXTENSIONS

| | | | | |
|---|---|---|---|---|
| 1. c | 8. a | 15. c | 22. d | 29. b |
| 2. d | 9. b | 16. b | 23. a | 30. a |
| 3. b | 10. d | 17. a | 24. c | 31. c |
| 4. b | 11. a | 18. b | 25. a | 32. d |
| 5. a | 12. c | 19. d | 26. b | 33. a |
| 6. d | 13. b | 20. c | 27. d | 34. c |
| 7. c | 14. d | 21. b | 28. c | 35. b |

## CHAPTER 19—WIGS AND HAIR ADDITIONS

| | | | | |
|---|---|---|---|---|
| 1. a | 7. b | 13. c | 19. d | 25. a |
| 2. c | 8. a | 14. b | 20. b | 26. b |
| 3. d | 9. d | 15. d | 21. c | 27. c |
| 4. b | 10. d | 16. b | 22. a | 28. b |
| 5. c | 11. c | 17. b | 23. c | 29. d |
| 6. a | 12. a | 18. a | 24. d | 30. a |

## CHAPTER 20—CHEMICAL TEXTURE SERVICES

| | | | | |
|---|---|---|---|---|
| 1. b | 14. a | 27. a | 40. d | 53. a |
| 2. c | 15. c | 28. c | 41. c | 54. c |
| 3. b | 16. b | 29. b | 42. b | 55. b |
| 4. d | 17. c | 30. a | 43. d | 56. d |
| 5. a | 18. a | 31. d | 44. a | 57. b |
| 6. b | 19. d | 32. a | 45. c | 58. a |
| 7. a | 20. a | 33. c | 46. a | 59. d |
| 8. a | 21. b | 34. b | 47. b | 60. c |
| 9. c | 22. a | 35. c | 48. a | 61. a |
| 10. b | 23. c | 36. d | 49. d | 62. b |
| 11. d | 24. d | 37. b | 50. c | 63. c |
| 12. a | 25. b | 38. a | 51. b | 64. d |
| 13. b | 26. d | 39. b | 52. d | 65. b |

## CHAPTER 21—HAIRCOLORING

| | | | | |
|---|---|---|---|---|
| 1. a | 15. b | 29. c | 43. b | 57. a |
| 2. c | 16. a | 30. a | 44. a | 58. d |
| 3. d | 17. b | 31. b | 45. d | 59. c |
| 4. b | 18. d | 32. d | 46. b | 60. b |
| 5. b | 19. c | 33. b | 47. c | 61. a |
| 6. a | 20. b | 34. c | 48. b | 62. d |
| 7. d | 21. a | 35. a | 49. d | 63. a |
| 8. c | 22. d | 36. b | 50. c | 64. b |
| 9. d | 23. a | 37. d | 51. c | 65. c |
| 10. a | 24. b | 38. b | 52. a | 66. b |
| 11. b | 25. c | 39. d | 53. a | 67. b |
| 12. c | 26. a | 40. c | 54. c | 68. d |
| 13. d | 27. c | 41. a | 55. d | 69. c |
| 14. d | 28. d | 42. d | 56. b | 70. a |

## CHAPTER 22—HAIR REMOVAL

| | | | | |
|---|---|---|---|---|
| 1. c | 6. a | 11. a | 16. a | 21. b |
| 2. b | 7. d | 12. b | 17. b | 22. d |
| 3. b | 8. a | 13. c | 18. d | 23. a |
| 4. a | 9. d | 14. d | 19. c | 24. c |
| 5. c | 10. c | 15. b | 20. a | 25. d |

## CHAPTER 23—FACIALS

| | | | | |
|---|---|---|---|---|
| 1. a | 11. d | 21. a | 31. c | 41. c |
| 2. b | 12. c | 22. c | 32. b | 42. a |
| 3. a | 13. d | 23. b | 33. a | 43. d |
| 4. d | 14. a | 24. d | 34. c | 44. b |
| 5. c | 15. c | 25. c | 35. d | 45. d |
| 6. b | 16. b | 26. b | 36. a | 46. a |
| 7. d | 17. b | 27. a | 37. b | 47. b |
| 8. a | 18. c | 28. a | 38. c | 48. c |
| 9. c | 19. a | 29. d | 39. b | 49. b |
| 10. a | 20. d | 30. b | 40. d | 50. d |

## CHAPTER 24—FACIAL MAKEUP

| | | | | |
|---|---|---|---|---|
| 1. b | 7. d | 13. d | 19. a | 25. b |
| 2. b | 8. c | 14. c | 20. b | 26. c |
| 3. d | 9. b | 15. a | 21. d | 27. d |
| 4. c | 10. a | 16. c | 22. c | 28. a |
| 5. a | 11. d | 17. b | 23. a | 29. c |
| 6. c | 12. b | 18. d | 24. b | 30. b |

## CHAPTER 25—MANICURING

| | | | | |
|---|---|---|---|---|
| 1. b | 8. c | 15. b | 22. d | 29. a |
| 2. a | 9. d | 16. d | 23. b | 30. b |
| 3. b | 10. b | 17. c | 24. a | 31. c |
| 4. c | 11. d | 18. d | 25. c | 32. b |
| 5. d | 12. a | 19. b | 26. d | 33. d |
| 6. c | 13. d | 20. c | 27. b | 34. a |
| 7. a | 14. c | 21. a | 28. d | 35. c |

## CHAPTER 26—PEDICURING

| | | | | |
|---|---|---|---|---|
| 1. c | 6. d | 11. a | 16. a | 21. a |
| 2. b | 7. a | 12. c | 17. c | 22. c |
| 3. c | 8. b | 13. d | 18. b | 23. d |
| 4. a | 9. c | 14. b | 19. b | 24. c |
| 5. d | 10. a | 15. d | 20. a | 25. d |

## CHAPTER 27—NAIL TIPS AND WRAPS

| | | | |
|---|---|---|---|
| 1. b | 6. c | 11. a | 16. b |
| 2. a | 7. d | 12. c | 17. d |
| 3. b | 8. b | 13. a | 18. b |
| 4. d | 9. d | 14. d | 19. c |
| 5. d | 10. b | 15. c | 20. a |

## CHAPTER 28—MONOMER LIQUID AND POLYMER POWDER NAIL ENHANCEMENTS

| | | | | |
|---|---|---|---|---|
| 1. b | 7. d | 13. b | 19. d | 25. c |
| 2. b | 8. b | 14. d | 20. a | 26. d |
| 3. a | 9. c | 15. b | 21. c | 27. a |
| 4. c | 10. a | 16. d | 22. a | 28. c |
| 5. d | 11. a | 17. a | 23. b | 29. b |
| 6. c | 12. c | 18. b | 24. d | 30. a |

## CHAPTER 29—UV GELS

| | | | |
|---|---|---|---|
| 1. c | 6. b | 11. b | 16. b |
| 2. b | 7. c | 12. a | 17. d |
| 3. d | 8. d | 13. d | 18. a |
| 4. a | 9. a | 14. c | 19. b |
| 5. c | 10. d | 15. c | 20. c |

## CHAPTER 30—SEEKING EMPLOYMENT

| | | | |
|---|---|---|---|
| 1. b | 6. d | 11. d | 16. d |
| 2. a | 7. a | 12. b | 17. c |
| 3. d | 8. b | 13. d | 18. a |
| 4. c | 9. c | 14. a | 19. b |
| 5. b | 10. c | 15. b | 20. a |

## CHAPTER 31—ON THE JOB

| | | | |
|---|---|---|---|
| 1. b | 6. b | 11. a | 16. a |
| 2. a | 7. a | 12. c | 17. c |
| 3. d | 8. b | 13. d | 18. d |
| 4. d | 9. d | 14. b | 19. b |
| 5. c | 10. c | 15. d | 20. a |

## CHAPTER 32—THE SALON BUSINESS

| | | | | |
|---|---|---|---|---|
| 1. d | 6. c | 11. c | 16. b | 21. c |
| 2. c | 7. b | 12. a | 17. d | 22. d |
| 3. b | 8. d | 13. c | 18. c | 23. b |
| 4. a | 9. a | 14. d | 19. a | 24. a |
| 5. d | 10. b | 15. a | 20. a | 25. d |